AF364241

PHARMACOGNOSY OF POWDERED CRUDE DRUGS

Prof. Dr. M. A. IYENGAR
14 HIG, Manipal
Former Professor & Head Dept. of Pharmacognosy
Manipal College of Pharmaceutical Sciences
Manipal University,
MANIPAL – 576 104
INDIA

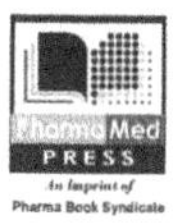 **PharmaMed Press**
An Imprint of Pharma Book Syndicate

A Unit of **BSP Books Pvt. Ltd.**

4-4-309/316, Giriraj Lane,
Sultan Bazar,
Hyderabad - 500 095.

PHARMACOGNOSY OF POWDERED CRUDE DRUGS

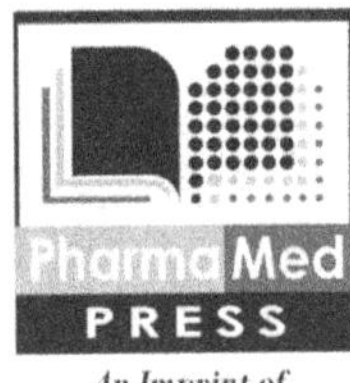

PharmaMed Press
An Imprint of Pharma Book Syndicate

A Unit of **BSP Books Pvt. Ltd.**

4-4-309/316, Giriraj Lane,
Sultan Bazar, Hyderabad - 500 095.

First Edition	:	1974
Second Edition	:	1980
Third Edition	:	1986
Fourth Edition	:	1993
Fifth Edition	:	1997
Sixth Edition	:	2001
Seventh Edition	:	2005
Eighth Edition	:	2007
Ninth Edition	:	2009
Tenth Edition	:	2011

2020 *Eighth Reprint*

ISBN : 978-93-89974-89-8

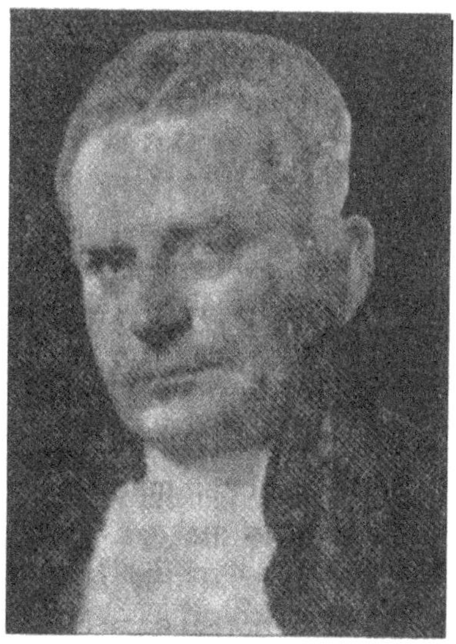

Dedicated with profound respects

to

one of the leading International Pharmacognosists
The Late Professor Dr. Dres. h.c. Ludwig Hörhammer

erstwhile Director

des

Instituts für Pharmazeutische Arzneimittellehre
der Universität München, München, West Germany

THE ACADEMY OF GENERAL EDUCATION
Manipal, Karnataka State

Dr. T. M. A. PAI, M.B.B.S.
President & Registrar

FOREWORD

A book dealing with the Pharmacognosy of Powdered Crude Drugs is a long felt necessity. As the desire to have indigenous drugs is growing in developing countries, all the available crude drugs have got to be identified and analysed.

A very strenuous effort has been made by the author to collect all the data that is necessary to make a publication of this type useful to the students of Pharmacy. Dr. Iyengar has shown that the subject that he has dealt with is not so easy as many people think. I have at random gone through some pages here and there and I have no hesitation in saying that the pharmacists will find this book very useful as it will enable them to carry on efforts in this direction for better and more productive purpose. This book which I understand is the first of its kind in India, gives correct and exact characters of identification stated in clear, simple language intelligible even to those who have no previous knowledge of this subject. Dr. Iyengar, on account of his studies both in India and also in Germany, has developed a new approach to make the subject presentable to students of Pharmacy.

I hope this book will be read widely.

1974

Dr. T. M. A. Pai

PREFACE

In June 1973, the author returned from Germany after a period of 7 years of stay, so as to take up the position of Associate Professor in Pharmacognosy, in the College of Pharmaceutical Sciences, Kasturba Medical College, Manipal. During day to day teaching, the author felt the dire necessity of a hand book on the study of powdered drugs which forms a major portion in Pharmacognosy course for the graduate students of Pharmacy all over India. In Germany and other western countries, there are atleast half-a-dozen different books available on this aspect. Thus, the 'germ of thought' was, 'then why not in India, for Indian students, of Indian drugs and by Indian authors ?' With this in mind, the author presents this booklet to the students of pharmacy all over the country, concerned researchers in the Drug Industries, Government Institutions of Health Ministry both the State and Central and Druggists dealing with indigenous drugs as well.

Thanks to Manipal, because it is this small village (Manipal-Fountain of knowledge) with a very high percentage of learned scholars, the prevailing educational atmosphere, unpolluted air and the challenging student community that gave impetus, initiative and inspiration to make this book a possibility.

Commerce is concomitant with adulteration and powdered crude drugs are no exception. This has been so since ages and shall continue for ever. Although this book is primarily meant for students, the author has not ignored the aspects on evaluation, adulteration, detection etc., over here. Thus it is hoped, that this hand book will not only be of immense use for the examinations but also to detect either deliberate or innocent adulteration which is a very important factor in Pharmacognosy.

There may be many omissions and commissions in this little monograph. The author sincerely wishes the kind co-operation of every reader in correcting them.

The diagrams have been drawn by Mr. S. Gopalkrishna Nayak, Demonstrator in the Department of Pharmacognosy here, whose kind help the author gratefully acknowledges at this juncture, but for which he could not have brought out this brochure within this short time. Grateful acknowledgements are also due to Padmashree Dr. T.M.A. Pai, President and Registrar, Academy of General Education, Manipal for his generous financial assistance in part and also for the foreword. Sincere thanks are also due to Professor Dr. A. Krishna Rao, Dean, Kasturba Medical College, Manipal for his constant encouragement. The author takes this opportunity to convey his heartfelt thanks to Prof. Dr. Ludwig Horharmmer,

Director des Instituts fur Pharmazeutische Arzneimittellehre der Universitaet, Muenchen, West Germany, to whom this book is also dedicated. The author is further indebted to The Alexander von Humboldt Foundation, Bonn-Bad Godesberg, West Germany, for their generous help not only during the author's tenure as a Humboldt Fellow, but even today in many different forms. Last but not least, sincere thanks are also due to Manipal Press Limited for kindly undertaking the job and executing the same in commendable manner within a short time. All care has been taken to revise and improve this edition.

July, 1980, Manipal

M. A. IYENGAR

3rd REPRINT

Every reprint of a book is a direct indication of the positive response of the student community. Majority of the features of the previous editions have been retained as no special comments, criticisms and suggestions have comeforth.

I gratefully acknowledge the continuous support and encouragement of Madam Dr. R. M. Captain, Ph.D. A.E.Ed. (Lond) of the Himalaya Drug Co. Bombay and of my colleague Shri S. G. K. Nayak.

Ganesh Chathurthi, September 1986   **M. A. IYENGAR**
Manipal

4th REPRINT

I thank all concerned for enabling me to bring out this 4th edition.

Shivarathri 1993   **M. A. IYENGAR**

5th REPRINT

I did not expect that the 5th reprint will see the light of the day. Thanks to all concerned.

Pongal, 1997   **M. A. IYENGAR**

6th REPRINT Ganesh Chathurthi, 2001

7th REPRINT 5th March, 2005

8th REPRINT Ganesh Chathurthi, 2007

9th REPRINT Ganesh Chathurthi, 2009

10th REPRINT December, 2011   **M. A. IYENGAR**

INTRODUCTION

Drugs have been dealt here on the basis of morphological classification. Roots are taken up first followed by rhizomes, stem barks (cortex), woods, leaves, flowers, fruits, seeds, entire organisms and starches almost corresponding to the natural phenomena of plant growth. And then, under each group the drugs are dealt in an alphabetical order. The drugs are prefixed intentionally with Latin terminology to familiarize the students in identifying the source without further preparation. For example, **Coriander** or **Clove** is very often problematic and puzzling to the students with regard to their sources. A student can overcome this by learning the names in complete like **Fructus Coriandri** or **Flores Caryophylli** which directly gives the morphological nature or source.

Drugs have been selected taking into consideration the Pharmacognosy course of different Institutions of Pharmacy in India. Although it would have been ideal to include all the I.P. drugs, for want of time and genuine drugs, the author has not been able to fulfil this expectation. On the other hand drugs like **Chamomile, Coffee** etc., have been included with different objectives in mind. Chamomile is used very often as a common household remedy in western countries and aptly it has been included not only in the different pharmacopoeias and syllabii of different Institutions and Universities but also in most of the pharmaceutical preparations. The author intends to publish another such manual on chromatography and drugs like **Coffee, Eucalyptus** etc., are introduced here with an idea to subject these also for chromatographic investigations.

Powdered drugs before use were sieved through 60 mesh. The mounting medium in general has been chloral hydrate, though water, iodine, phloroglucin +HCL (1+1), lactophenol etc., were also employed for the study, where necessary, Majority of the tissues were studied and drawn directly from the microscope. Place of study has been the Pharmacognosy Laboratory of the College of Pharmaceutical Sciences, Kasturba Medical College, Manipal. Powders with similar or overlapping characters leading to confusion in identification have been emphasized where necessary with an **'attention'** mark and at time proper clues have been provided for clarification. Further, only diagnostic characteristics with which one can identify a drug are mentioned. Characters common to many drugs are deliberately omitted. So also, the routine macroscopic observations like the colour, nature, taste and odour, unless they have something special, are not given, as they do not lead one anywhere in identifying powders in a mixture. The sequence of the characteristics are according to their importance in identification. The numbers of identifying characters correspond to the numbers of diagrams.

Mixture in examinations usually consists of 2 to 4 powdered drugs. This has to be identified and analysed giving reasons. To illustrate, in a mixture like lignum **Santalum,** folia **Vasaka** and fructus **Capsicum,** the individual components are identified under the following proforma: The given mixture contains lignum **Santalum** because of the following reasons (all the characters are to be given as in the text here). The second powder appears to be folia **Vasaka** for the reasons given below (refer text). The third component is fructus **Capsicum** on the basis of the following characters (See text). Needless to mention here the reasons are to be well supported by appropriate diagrams.

In order to get optimum benefit the student is advised to use this book regularly during his practical study.

How to mount the powdered drugs for microscopic examination ?

For microscopic examination, one prepares invariably three slides; one in Chloral hydrate, one in water and one in Phloroglucinol+HCl.

A judicious quantity of powder is taken on a glass slide to which are added a few drops of chloral hydrate and is heated for 1 – 2 min. after placing a cover slip. Care however is to be taken to avoid air bubbles and to see that there is sufficient chloral hydrate under the coverslip. Excess of Chloral hydrate outside the coverslip is to be withdrawn using a blotting paper. Chloral hydrate is used to clear the tissues and to bring in clarity of the view.

In order to observe strach grains, mount the powder in water. Bring 1 to 2 drops of dil. iodine in contact with the edge of the cover slip. Starch grains appear light blue in colour.

Lignified tissues are to be confirmed after staining. To the powder cleared as above a few drops of mixture of 1:1 Phloroglucinol+Con. HCl are added and after 3 to 4 minutes, it is finally mounted in Chloral hydrate/glycerine. Care is to be taken to avoid the acid vapours from coming into contact with the microscopic objectives.

CONTENTS

TUBERA ACONITI (ACONITE)

Aconitum species   Ranunculaceae

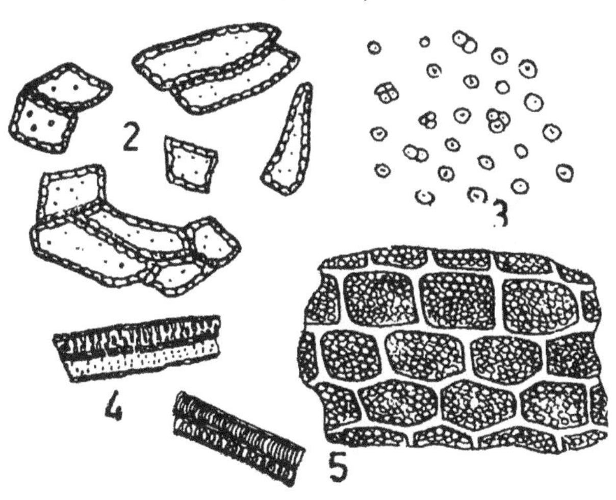

Identifying Characters

1. **Taste:** persistent tingling sensation followed by numbness.

2. **Stone cells:** oval to quadratic, evenly thickened, lignified, with simple pits and large lumina.

3. **Starch granules:** abundant, both simple and compound (2-6 components) and each measures somewhere between 3 and 30 microns in diameter.

4. **Tracheal elements:** fragments of vessels possessing all kinds of thickenings like – spiral, annular, reticulate, though slit like pitted thickenings predominate.

5. **Parenchyma:** thick walled isodiametric cells fully loaded with starch grains.

RADIX BELLADONNAE

Atropa belladonna L.   Solanaceae

A. acuminata Royle ex Lindley

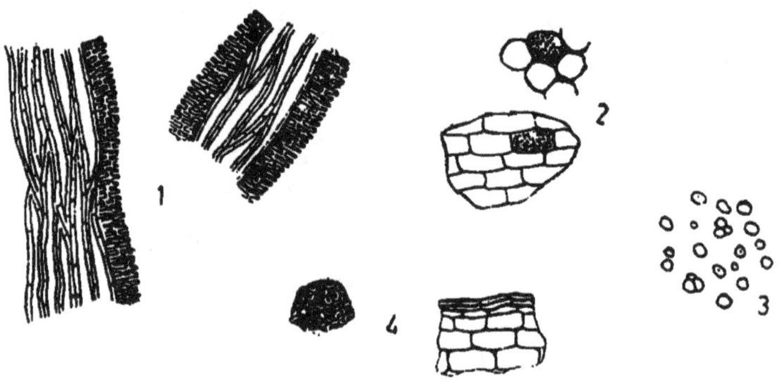

Identifying Characters

1. **Wood elements:** xylem vessels and fibres inter-lock with each other to form a spindle shaped structure which is characteristic to this root.

2. **Calcium oxalate:** sandy balls of the calcium oxalate in the cortical cells.

3. **Starch granules:** both simple and compound (2-4 components), spherical to round with an indistinct hilum.

4. **Cork:** cell walls of the cork are thickened.

RADIX GENTIAN

Gentiana lutea L.   Gentianaceae

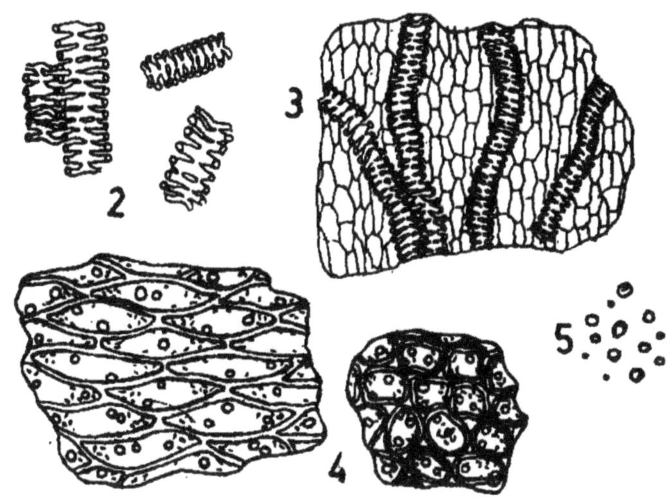

Identifying Characters

1. **Taste:** persistently bitter.

2. **Vessels:** well developed wide vessels with reticulate thickening.
   Attention – Rhizma **Podophylli**.

3. **Vascular elements:** characteristic pattern or design of the
   'run-way' of the vascular elements.

4. **Parenchyma:** thick walled cells containing oil globules and
   minute acicular raphides.

5. **Starch grains:** small, simple and not many.

RADIX IPECAC

Cephaelis ipecacuanha (Brot). A Rich   Rubiaceae

C. acuminata Karsten.

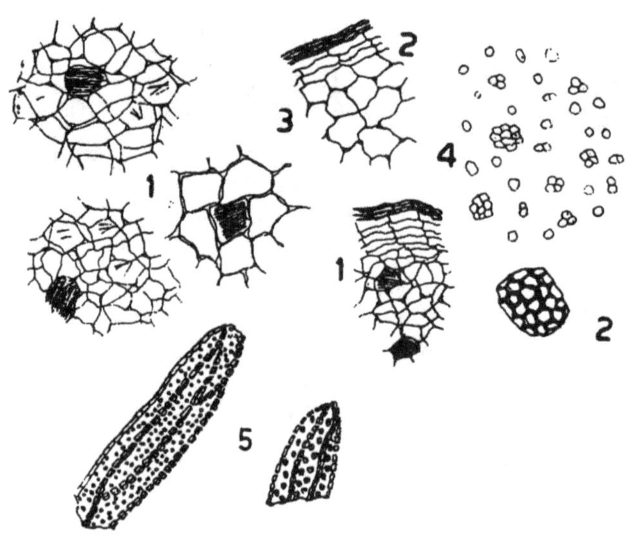

Identifying Characters

1. **Acicular raphides:** cortical parenchyma containing acicular raphides either in bundles or scattered all over.

2. **Cork:** polygonal, more or less isodiametric in surface view. Side view of cork with parenchyma is also seen very often.

3. **Parenchyma:** cortical parenchyma consisting of thin walled polyhedral cells with intercellular spaces.

4. **Starch granules:** compound granules large in number; individual granule measures not more than 15 microns. Some grains show prominent hilum.

5. **Trachea and Tracheids:** small with linear pits (magnified).

RADIX LICORICE

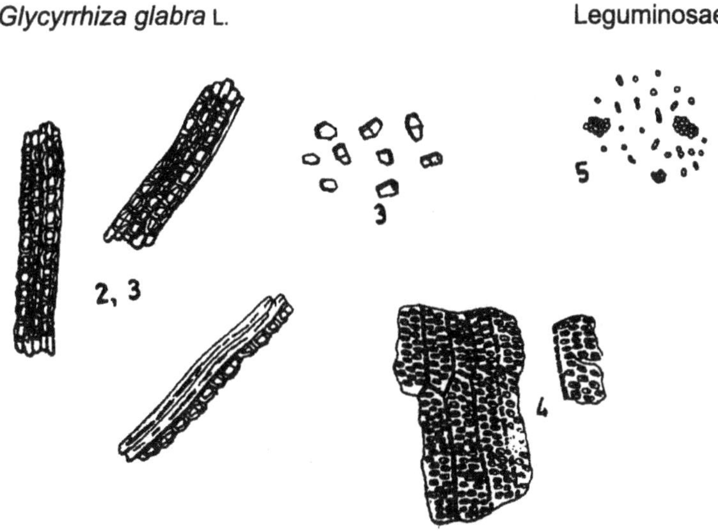

Identifying Characters

1. **Taste:** sweet.

2. **Fibres:** yellow coloured fibres in bundles of about 10-15; the tips of the bundles appear fringed like that of an 'electric cable'.

3. **Calcium oxalate:** parenchymatous sheath of small parenchymatous cells (crystal sheath), each containing a single prism of calcium oxalate, encircle the above fibres; scattered prisms are also seen (mostly twin prisms).

   Attention: Cortex **Cascara**, Cortex **Quillaia** and Folia Senna.

4. **Wood elements:** vessels large, with numerous bordered pits.

5. **Starch granules:** both simple (oval to elongated) and compound (not many), minute.

RADIX RAUWOLFIA

Rauwolfia serpentina Bentham.   Apocynaceae

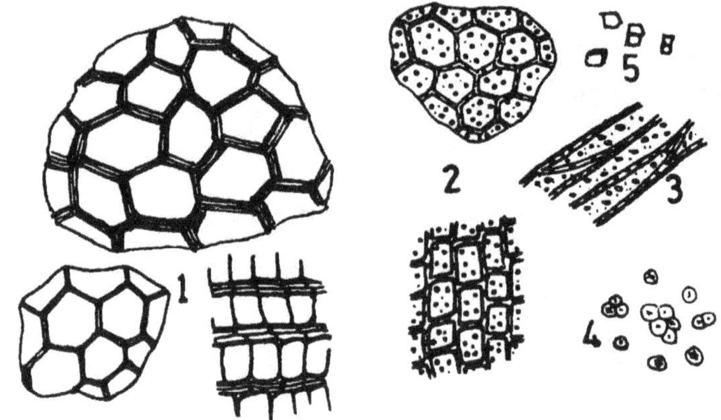

Identifying Characters

1. **Cork:** stratified cork in several layers (some lignified) appearing like 'benzene' rings, in surface view.

2. **Parenchyma:** pitted and lignified parenchymatous cells of the xylem parenchyma and medullary ray cells.

3. **Wood elements:** vessels few, long and with oblique end walls and perforations.

4. **Starch granules:** largely simple but compound ones are also known to occur. Granules are fairly large, possessing a distinct hilum in the form of a 'star' or a 'split'.

5. **Calcium oxalate:** crystals in the form of prisms but not many in number.

RHIZOMA CURCUMAE

Curcuma longa L.   Zingiberaceae

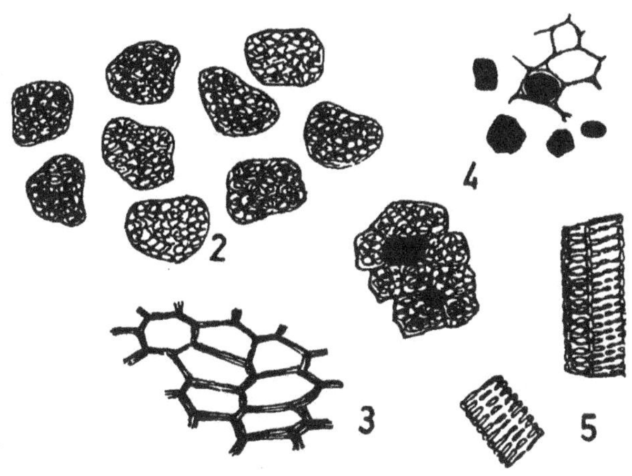

Identifying Characters

1. **Naked eye observation:** the slide takes a deep yellow colour on treatment with cold Chloral hydrate.

2. **Starch granules:** appear in big rounded pasty masses with yellowish tinge.

3. **Cork:** the cork cells show striations in surface view.

4. **Oleoresin cells:** scattered all over with brownish contents.

5. **Wood elements:** well developed wide vessels with reticulate and spiral thickenings.

RHIZOMA RHEI (RHUBARB)

Rheum palmatum L.   Polygonaceae

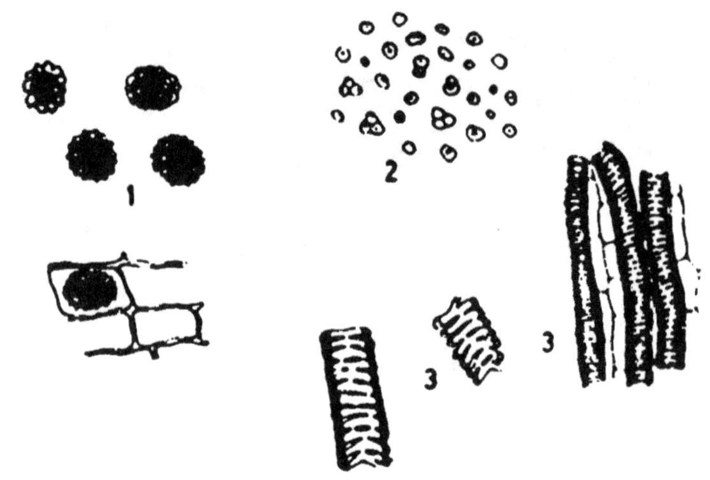

Identifying Characters

1. **Calcium oxalate crystals:** cluster crystals as big as 100 microns in diameter with well defined and pointed corners; many in number and scattered all over.

2. **Starch granules:** sphaeroidal or angular in shape, both simple and compound (2-5) and show a distinct central hilum.

3. **Wood elements:** vessels are very wide, reticulately thickened and do not show any lignin reaction with the usual Phloroglucin+HCl.

4. **Chemical test:** powder on treatment with caustic potash gives blood red colouration.

RHIZOMA ZINGIBERIS (GINGER)

Zingiber officinale Roscoe.   Zingiberaceae

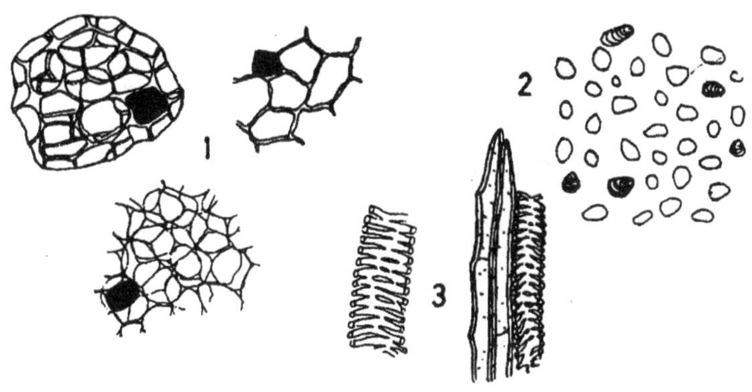

Identifying Characters

Odour: Pleasant and aromatic

Taste: Pungent

1. **Parenchyma:** some of the cells contain yellow-brown oleoresinous bodies which occur either in fragments or as droplets.

2. **Starch grains:** characteristic, abundant, simple, ovoid or sack shaped, 5 to 60 microns in length and have a distinct eccentric hilum.

3. **Fibres and Vessels:** septate fibres in groups associated with vessels, fibres mostly non-lignified.

PODOPHYLLI
(INDIAN PODOPHYLLUM)

Podophyllum emodi Wall.   Berberidaceae

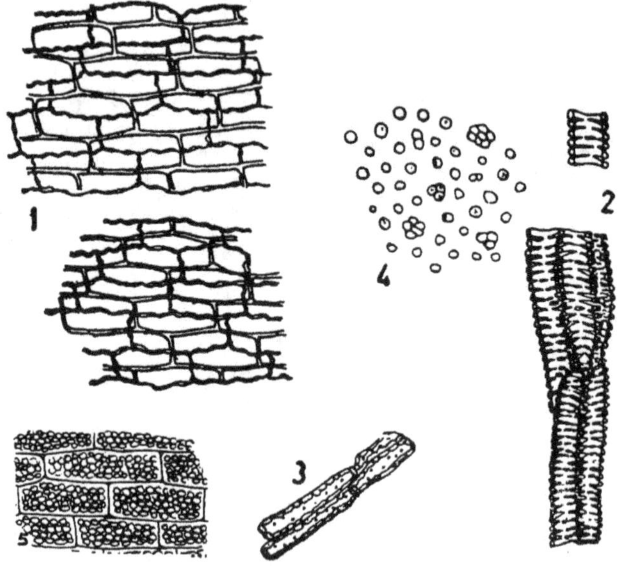

Identifying Characters

1. **Epiblema x Exodermis:** abundant fragments of the outer layer of the roots (epiblema) in association with exodermis (wavy walls).

2. **Wood elements:** large number of vessels, either entire or fragments of the same showing reticulate thickening.

   Attention: Radix **Gentian.**

3. **Sclereids:** in groups, uniformly thickened and rectangular in shape (very rare).

4. **Starch granules:** abundant, simple (spherical to ovoid) and compound (3-8).

5. **Parenchyma:** Parenchyma with fully loaded starch grains.

VALERIAN

Valeriana Wallichii DC   Valerianaceae

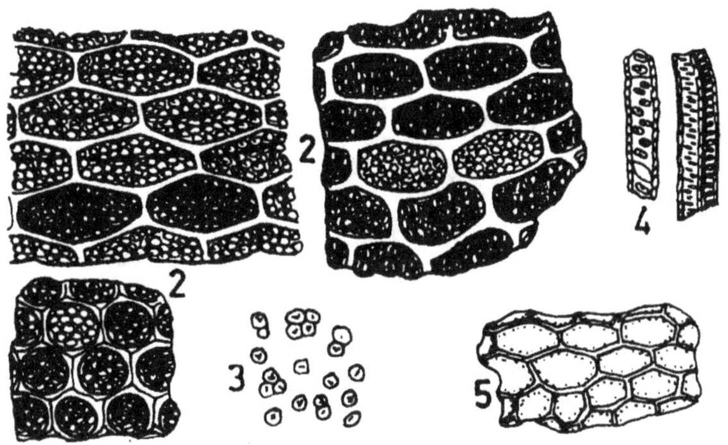

Identifying Characters

1. **Odour:** very characteristic.

2. **Parenchyma:** typical parenchymatous cells which are either rounded or elongated, yellowish and are full of starch grains. Some of the parenchymatous cells are opalescent.

3. **Starch granules:** rounded, mostly simple, compound one containing 2-4 components; hilum though indistinct, may be seen as a cleft.

4. **Wood elements:** vessels with bordered pits, scalariform and spiral thickenings.

5. **Cork:** lignified large polygonal cells from the periderm of rhizome.

CORTEX ASHOKA

Saraca indica L. Leguminosae

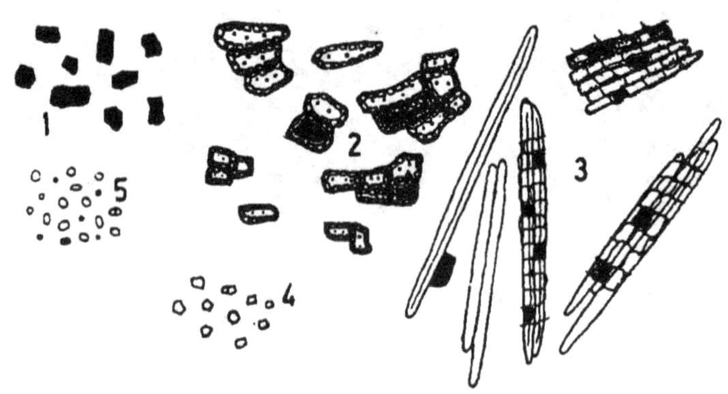

Identifying Characters

1. **Brown masses:** abundant yellowish brown masses characterize the slide.

2. **Stone cell:** occur in three different forms – linear, conical and rectangular, all highly pitted including their walls; often in groups. At times they do contain some brownish matter.

3. **Phloem fibres:** occur lengthwise in groups of 3 to 5. Between the fibres are seen the above mentioned brown masses adhering to the fibres.

4. **Calcium oxalate:** in the form of small prisms, rather not so common.

5. **Starch:** simple, round, rarely compound and not characteristic.

CORTEX CASCARA

Rhamnus purshiana DC.   Rhamnaceae

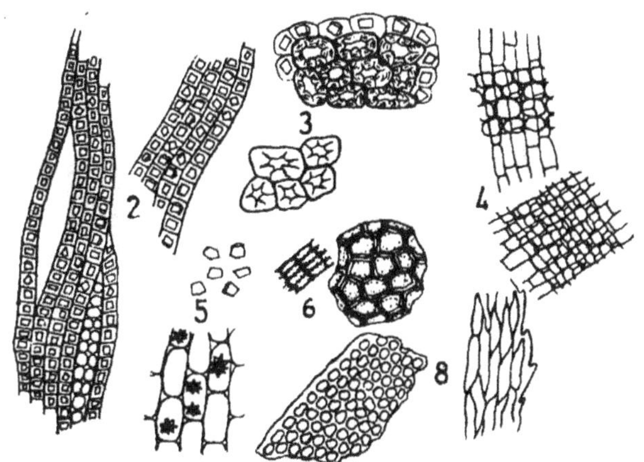

Identifying Characters

1. **Taste:** nauseous, bitter and persistent.
2. **Phloem fibres:** fragments or entire pieces of fibres which are encircled by a parenchymatous sheath of cells possessing rows of prisms of calcium oxalate. This tissue appears yellow in a Chloral hydrate mount (**Attention**: Folia **Senna**, Cortex **Quillaia** and Radix **Licorice**.)
3. **Stone cells:** in groups, rounded and yellow; groups of sclereids or stone cells are surrounded by imperfect crystal sheath. Some stone cells are tangentially elongated with uniformly thickened walls.
4. **Medullary ray cells x phloem paranchyma:** numerous fragments of phloem tissue crossing medullary ray cells at right angles.
5. **Calcium oxalate crystals:** prisms and clusters of calcium oxalate in the cortical parenchyma and as well free in the powder.
6. **Cork:** occasional fragments of cork with thin walled cells, polygonal in surface view and containing brownish matter.
7. **Chemical test:** 1. Yellow colour is seen in a Chloral hydrate preparation. 2. With KOH, the preparation turns red (anthraquinone).
8. Foreign elements like fragments of lichens and moss may also appear in powder.

CORTEX CASSIA

Cinnamomum cassia Blume   Lauraceae

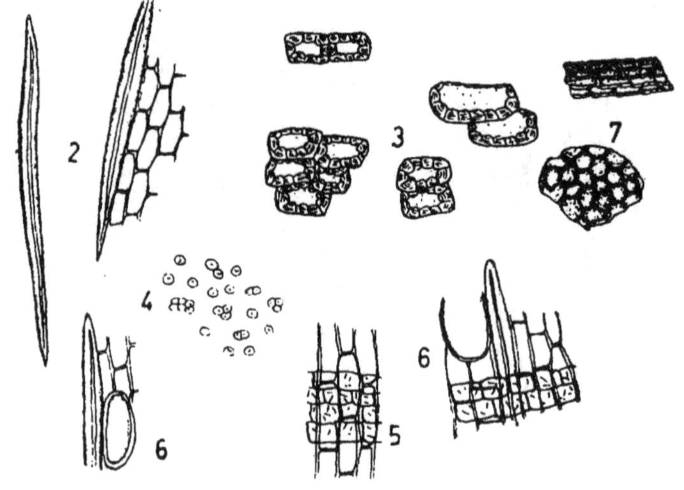

Identifying Characters

1. **Odour:** the typical pleasant aroma.

2. **Fibres:** thin, narrow, pointed and isolated bast fibres measure 250-700 microns in length and 15-45 microns in breadth.

3. **Stone cells:** in groups, rectangular (appears as 'U' shaped as one wall is not thickened) and pitted.

4. **Starch:** abundant starch and the grains measure upto 20 microns.

5. **Calcium oxalate:** is represented in the form of minute needles (acicular raphides) in medullary ray cells and phloem parenchyma.

6. **Oil cells:** big and isolated.

7. **Cork:** occasional fragments.

CORTEX CINNAMOMI

Cinnamomum zeylanicum Blume   Lauraceae

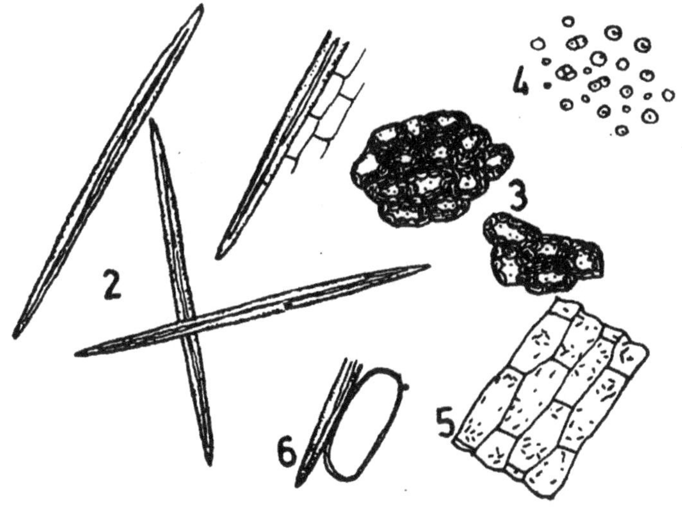

Identifying Characters

1. **Odour:** the typical sweet fragrance.

2. **Fibres:** isolated bast fibres measure 250-600 microns in length and 15-30 microns in breadth.

3. **Stone cells:** almost 'U' shaped as one wall is thinner than the other three.

4. **Starch grains:** abundant starch which does not measure more than 10 microns.

5. **Calcium oxalate crystals:** presence of small acicular raphides in the parenchyma.

6. **Oil cells:** big and isolated.

7. **Cork:** SHOULD NOT BE PRESENT.

CORTEX CINCHONA

Cinchona calisaya Weddell   Rubiaceae
C. ledgeriana Moens
C. officinalis L.
C. succirubra Pavon

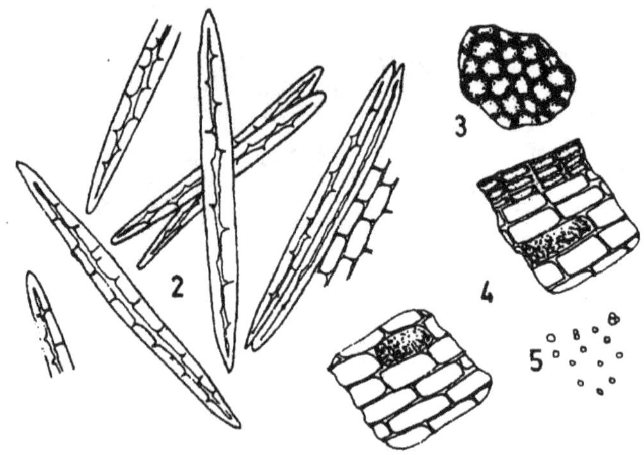

Identifying Characters

1. **Taste:** astringent and bitter.

2. **Fibres:** phloem fibres or bast fibres, numerous either entire or in fragments, spindle shaped, yellowish, thick walled, strongly lignified, porous walls having simple pores or branched pores and measure around 500 – 1350 microns in length and 50 – 130 microns in width.

3. **Cork:** typical thin walled cork cells which appear reddish brown in colour.

4. **Calcium oxalate crystals:** microsphenoidal crystals in dark coloured parenchyma.

5. **Starch grains:** minute, both simple and compound (2-5) and the individual grains measure 3 to 10 microns in diameter.

6. **Negative observations:** absence of cluster crystals and stone cells.

7. **Test:** powdered Cinchona when heated in a dry test tube in a slanting position, purple condensation is seen on the upper side of the test tube.

CORTEX KURCHI

Holarrhena antidysenterica Wall   Apocynaceae

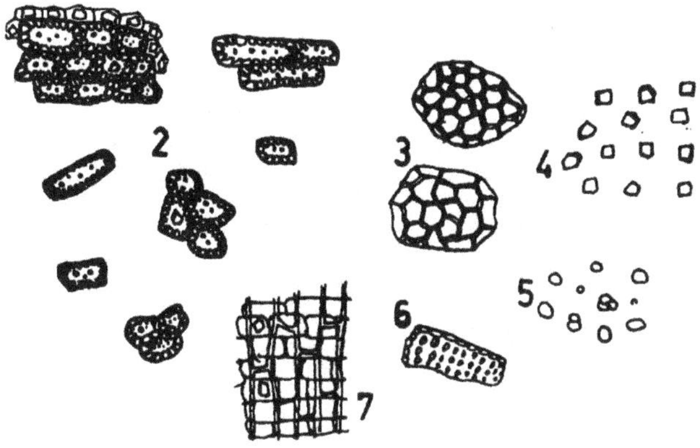

Identifying Characters

1. **Taste:** bitter.

2. **Stone cells:** in groups, rectangular to elongated (individual ones), walls striated and have pitted thickenings and some contain prisms in them.

3. **Cork cells:** thin walled, some colourless and others brown.

4. **Calcium oxalate crystals:** present in the form of prisms, scattered all over in the powder.

5. **Starch grains:** few and simple.

6. **Wood elements:** these should not appear in the powder as a rule but some wood elements may creep in here.

7. **Medullary rays:** phloem parenchyma traverse the medullary rays at right angles though such pieces are not seen many in number.

Note: Absence of phloem fibres.

CORTEX QUILLAIA

Quillaia saponaria Molina   Rosaceae

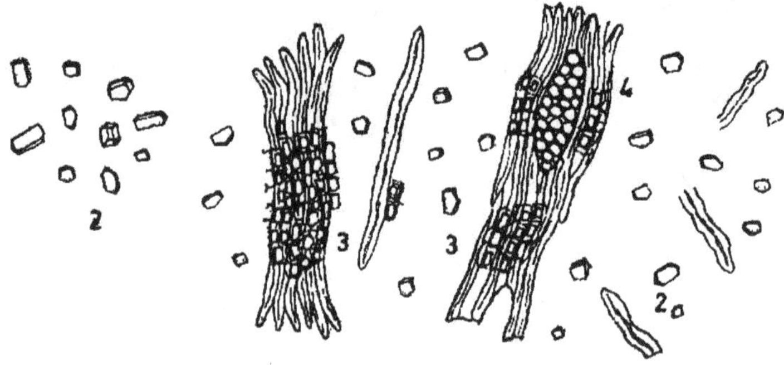

Identifying Characters

1. **Sternutatory action:** powder irritates the nostril and produces prolonged sneezing.

2. **Calcium oxalate crystals:** large number of big elongated prisms either entire or in fragments; some may also appear cubical in form; prisms are found scattered all over.

3. **Fibres:** phloem fibres appear in groups, individual fibre is thick, slender, coarse and may appear either entire or in fragments. Some of the parenchymatous cells surrounding the groups of fibres contain calcium oxalate crystals arranged in rows.

   Attention: Folia **Senna**, Cortex **Cascara**, Radix **Licorice**.

4. **Medullary ray cells:** some portions of tissues in the powder may reveal the width and height of medullary ray cells.

5. **Test for saponins:** when shaken with water a copious persistent froth is formed.

LIGNUM QUASSIA (QUASSIA WOOD)

Picrasma quassioides Benth

Simarubaceae

or

Picroena quassioides Benth

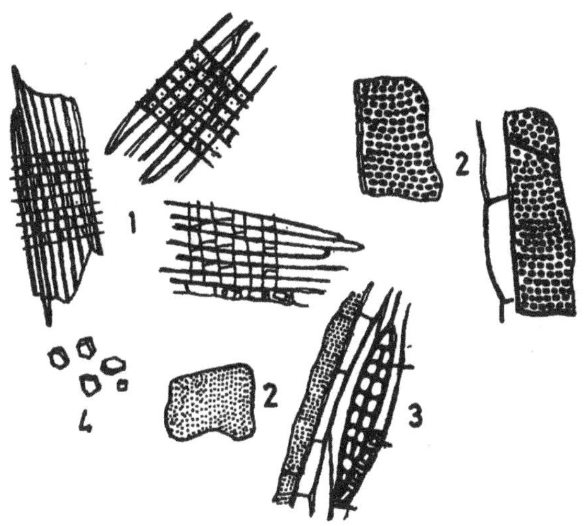

Identifying Characters

Taste: extremely bitter even in minute quantities.

1. **Wood elements:** abundant fragments of xylem fibres crossing at right angles the medullary ray cells.

2. **Wood elements:** xylem vessels with numerous bordered pitted thickening.

3. **Medullary ray cells:** very prominent; in tangential longitudinal view their heights can be measured.

4. **Calcium oxalate:** present in the form of prisms in the cells of wood parenchyma, but very rare.

Note: Being wood, all tissues are lignified.

LIGNUM SANTALUM (SANDAL WOOD)

Santalum album. L   Santalaceae

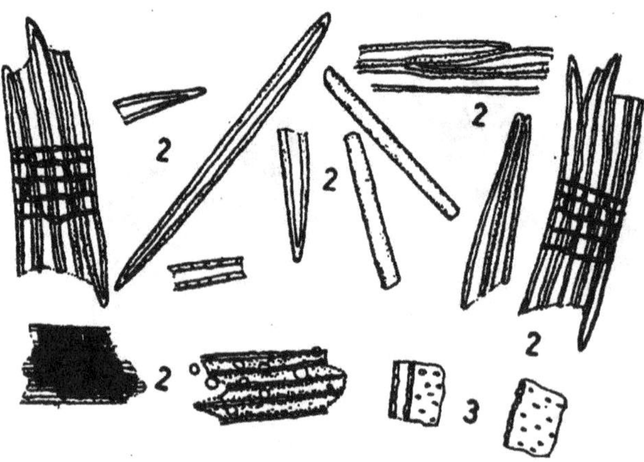

Identifying Characters

1. **Aroma:** very characteristic.

2. **Xylem Fibres:** large number of thick walled, elongated fibres (mostly in groups) which are at times traversed at right angles by thick walled characteristic medullary ray cells. Oil drops appear to be freely distributed in the wood fibres. Some brownish matter is also seen in most of the wood elements. The walls of a few fibres show pitted thickening. Pieces of isolated, thin walled and unpitted fibres are also seen here and there.

3. **Vessels:** fragments of xylem vessels are very wide and show a few bordered pits (not many).

Note: Being wood, all tissues are lignified.

FOLIA BELLADONNAE

Atropa belladonna L.   Solanaceae

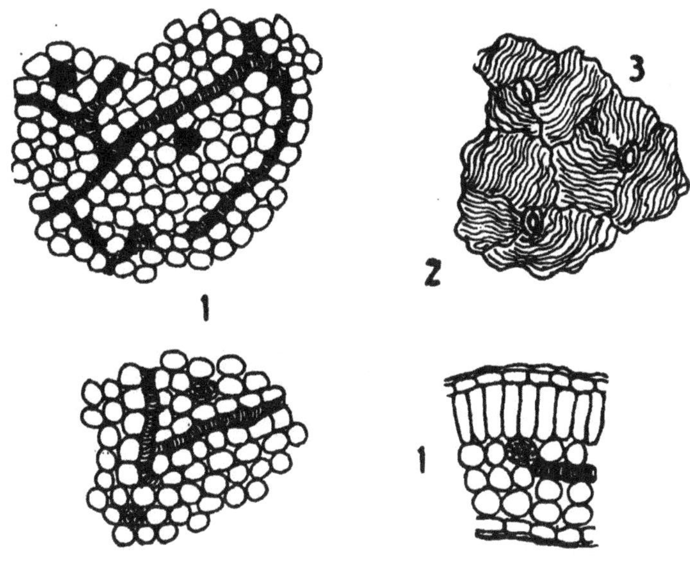

Identifying Characters

1. **Calcium oxalate crystals:** fragments of mesophyll tissue containing sandy balls particularly in the vicinity of vascular strands.

2. **Stomata:** anisocytic or cruciferous type meaning thereby that the stomal pore is surrounded by 3 epidermal cells of which one is invariably smaller than the other two.

3. **Epidermal cells:** walls of the epidermal cells are wavy and striations are seen on the cuticle.

4. **Trichomes:** rare but both covering and glandular trichomes appear to occur (could not be confirmed in the sample studied here).

FOLIA DIGITALIS

Digitalis purpurea L.   Scrophulariaceae

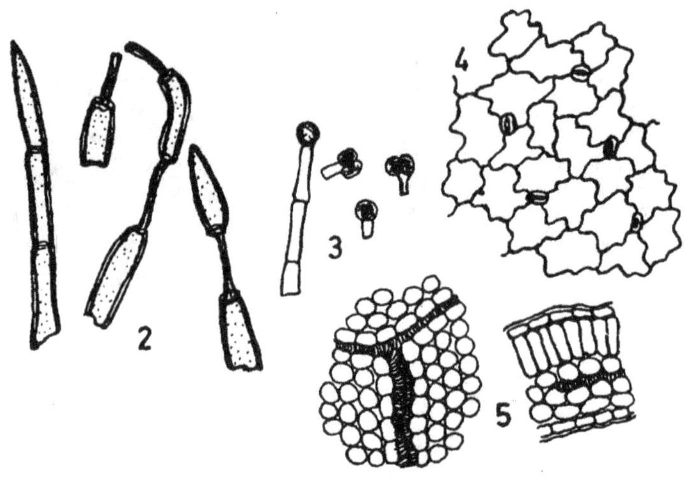

Identifying Characters

1. **Trichomes:** both covering and glandular, sometimes in fragments.

2. **Covering trichomes:** multicellular (3-5 celled) with blunt tips and finely warty. Certain cells of the trichomes are often collapsed leaving behind only the cell walls.
   Attention: Folia **Hyoscyamus**.

3. **Glandular trichomes:** less numerous, with both unicellular and multicellular stalk and a bicellular or multicellular terminal gland.

4. **Stomata:** Anomocytic or Ranunculaceous type.

5. **Negative character:** absence of calcium oxalate crystals.

FOLIA DIGITALIS

Digitalis lanata Ehrh   Scrophulariaceae

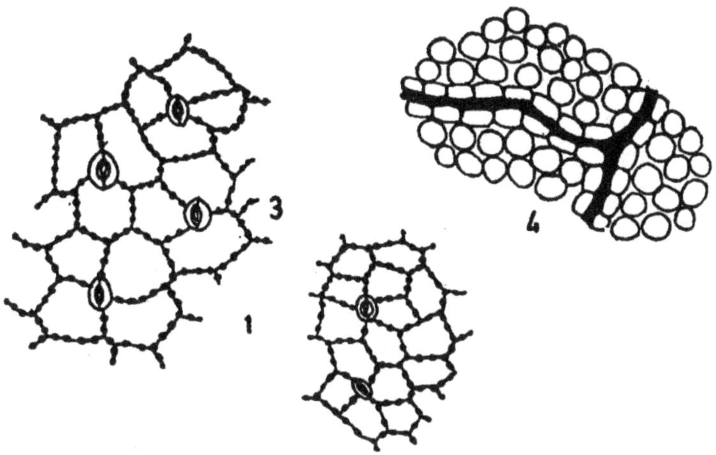

Identifying Characters

1. **Epidermal cells:** with irregularly beaded walls as seen in surface view.

2. **Stomata:** numerous anomocytic or Ranunculaceous stomata meaning thereby that the cells surrounding the stomatal pores are irregularly arranged and cannot be differentiated from other epidermal cells.

3. **Trichomes:** very rare, covering trichomes 10-14 celled and glandular trichomes with unicellular stalks and bicellular heads or with unicellular heads and 2-8 celled uniseriate stalks (not drawn here for obvious reasons).

4. **Negative character:** absence of calcium oxalate crystals.

FOLIA EUCALYPTI

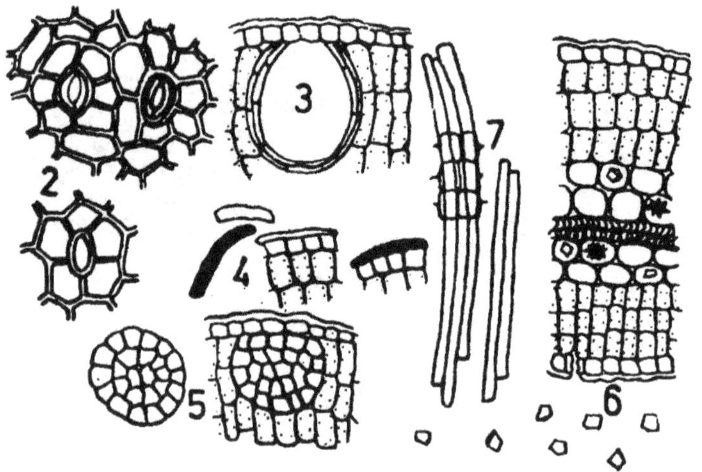

Identifying Characters

1. **Odour:** characteristic aroma.

2. **Epidermal cells:** polygonal epidermal cells with numerous, well developed, prominent and sunken stomata (anomocytic or Ranunculaceous type).

3. **Oil glands:** large secretory oil glands either entire or in fragments.

4. **Cuticle:** thick, shining, hyaline and curved fragments of cuticle.

5. **Cork:** fragments of cork tumors or proliferations.

6. **Calcium oxalate crystals:** both prisms and cluster crystals, but the latter less frequent.

7. **Fibre:** well developed sclerenchymatous fibres from the vascular bundle region.

FOLIA HYOSCYAMUS

Iyoscyamus niger L.　　　　　　　　　　Solanaceae

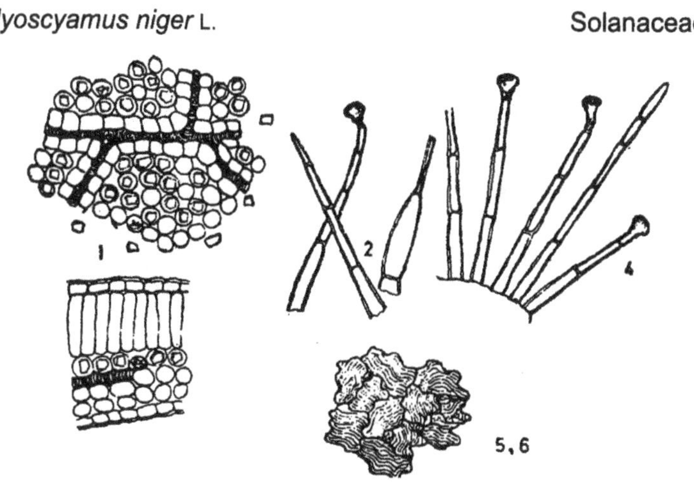

Identifying Characters

1. **Calcium oxalate prisms:** fragments of mesophyll tissue containing prisms in the vicinity of vascular strands, are seen good many in number. Cells adjacent to vascular strands do not contain calcium oxalate prisms.

2. **Trichomes:** both covering trichomes and glandular trichomes are present in abundance.

3. **Covering trichomes:** numerous, simple, uniseriate with nearly smooth surface.

4. **Glandular trichomes:** also numerous, either fragments or entire with 2-6 celled uniseriate stalk and with a large oval multicellular head.

5. **Stomata:** Cruciferous or Anisocytic type (for meaning refer Folia **Belladonna**).

6. **Epidermal cells:** with sinuous walls and with striated cuticle **Attention**: As some cells of the trichomes collapse as in that of Folia **Digitalis**, all care should be taken in studying other characters. Further, Folia **Stramonium** contains crystal-layer made of only cluster crystals whereas Folia **Hyoscyamus** (crystal-layer) contains largely prisms and at times cluster crystals as well.

FOLIA MENTHA

Mentha piperita L.　　　　　　　　　　　　　　Labiatae

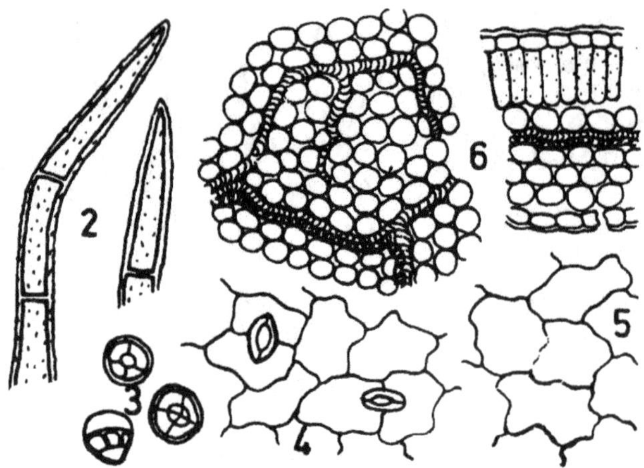

Identifying Characters

1. **Trichomes:** both covering and glandular.

2. **Covering trichomes:** thick, rugged, coarse, uniseriate with many cells.

3. **Glandular trichomes:** with unicellular stalk and a head with 1-8 cells (often yellow in colour).

4. **Stomata:** Caryophyllaceous or Diacytic type meaning thereby the two subsidiary cells are at right angles to the stomal pore (other examples of this type are – Folia **Vasaka** and Herba **Kalmegh**).

5. **Epidermis:** cells with wavy margin.

6. **Negative character:** absence of calcium oxalate crystals in the mesophyll tissue.

FOLIA SENNA

Cassia angustifolia Vahl   Leguminosae

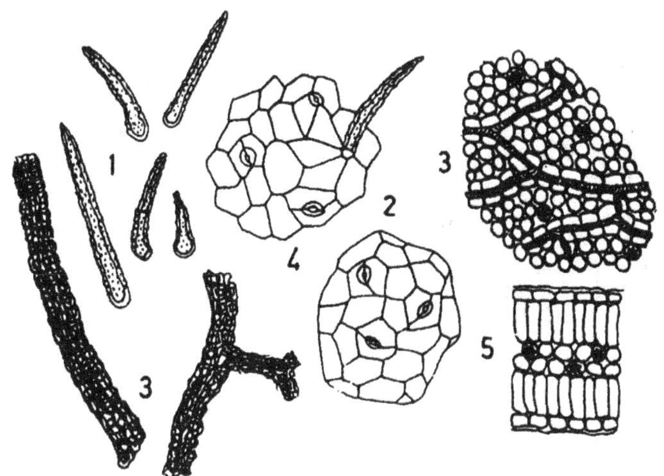

Identifying Characters

1. **Trichomes:** only covering type, short, thick, unicellular, warty and frequently curved near the base.

2. **Stomata:** Rubiaceous or paracytic type meaning thereby the two subsidiary cells are parallel to the stomal pore.

3. **Calcium oxalate:** occurring as cluster crystals in the cells of the mesophyll and as prisms in a sheath of cells around the fibres and as well freely distributed in powder.

   Attention: Cortex **Cascara**, Cortex **Quillaia**, Radix **Licorice**.

4. **Epidermis:** with polygonal epidermal cells in surface view.

5. **Mesophyll:** fragments of leaf showing isobilateral arrangement.

FOLIA STRAMONII

Datura stramonium L.   Solanaceae

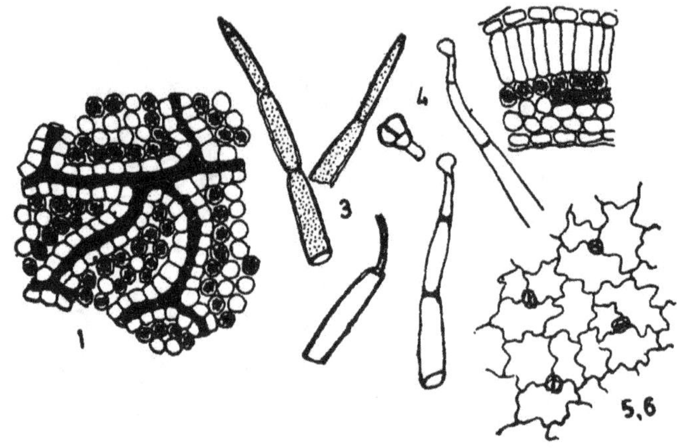

Identifying Characters

1. **Calcium oxalate crystals:** fragments of mesophyll tissue containing cluster crystals around vascular strands one in each cell. The cells adjacent to vascular strands do not contain any crystals.

2. **Trichomes:** both covering and glandular type.

3. **Covering trichomes:** warty, many celled, sometimes in fragments.

4. **Glandular trichomes:** with multicellular or unicellular head on a short stalk of 2 or more cells.

5. **Stomata:** Cruciferous or Anisocytic type.

6. **Epidermis:** cells with more or less sinuous walls and with smooth cuticle.

Attention: Folia **Hyoscyamus** contains well marked crystal-layer made of more prisms and less of cluster crystals. Trichomes with collapsed cells like that of Folia **Digitalis** and Folia **Hyoscyamus** are seen here too, though not characteristic but certainly confusing.

FOLIA THEAE (TEA)

Camellia sinesis (L.) O. Ktze   *Theaceae*

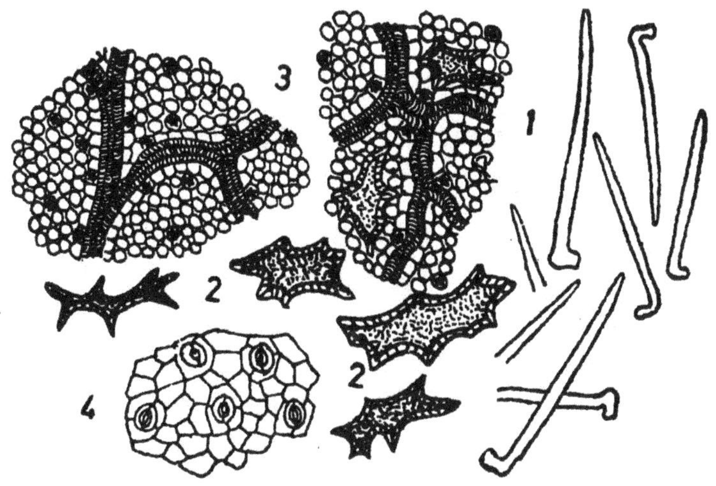

Identifying Characters

1. **Trichomes:** only covering type, unicellular, thick walled, lignified, pointed at one end and has a base like that of hockey stick.

2. **Sclereids:** numerous, large, irregular in form, lignified (sclerenchymatous idioblasts).

3. **Calcium oxalate:** cluster crystals scattered, throughout in the mesophyll tissue.

4. **Stomata:** Cruciferous or Anisocytic type.

FOLIA VASAKA

Adhatoda vasica Nees   Acanthaceae

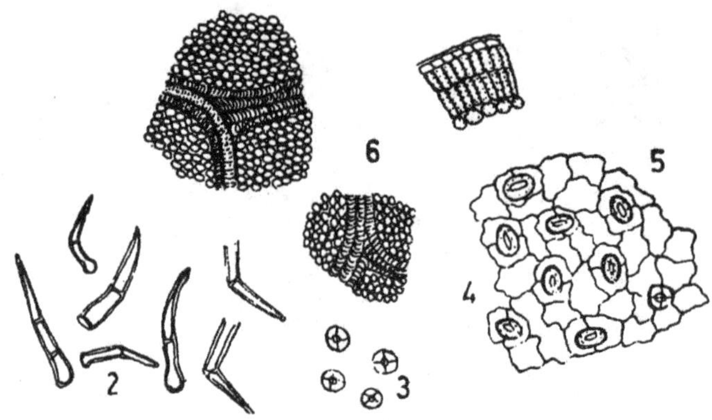

Identifying Characters

1. **Trichomes:** both covering and glandular type.

2. **Covering trichomes:** thick walled, minute, 2 - 4 celled (knee shaped) trichomes.

3. **Glandular trichomes:** sessile with quadricellular heads.

4. **Stomata:** Caryophyllaceous or Diacytic type (for meaning and other examples refer Folia **Mentha** and Herba **Kalmegh**).

5. **Epidermis:** cells with wavy outline.

6. **Negative characters:** absence of calcium oxalate crystals of any sort.

BULBUS SCILLAE (SQUILL)

Urginea indica Kunth   Liliaceae

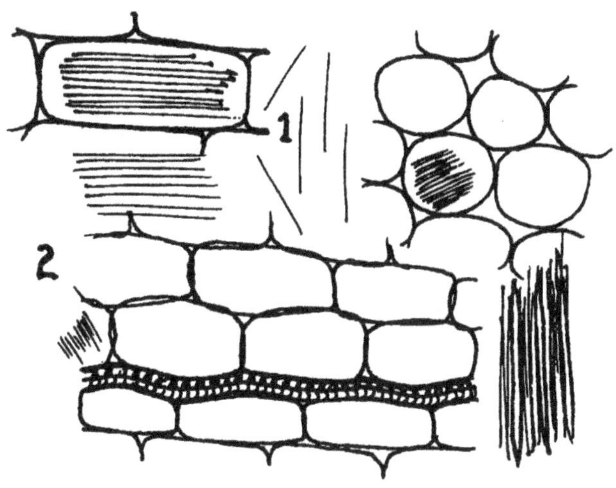

Identifying Characters

1. **Acicular raphides:** large number of acicular raphides mostly in bundles measuring around 1000 microns in length and around 20 microns in width, scattered all over in parenchyma.

   Attention: Radix **Ipecac**.

2. **Parenchyma:** colourless and large parenchymatous tissue containing vascular elements.

3. **Negative characters:** absence of trichomes, abundant starch grains, cluster crystals and prisms.

4. **Chemical test:**
   1. Mucilage does not turn pink with Ruthenium Red but stains with corallin soda soln.
   2. With Iodine water mucilage turns reddish purple.

FLORES CARYOPHYLLI

Syzygium aromaticum (L) Merill et. L. M. Perry

(*Eugenia caryophyllata* Thumb) Myrtaceae

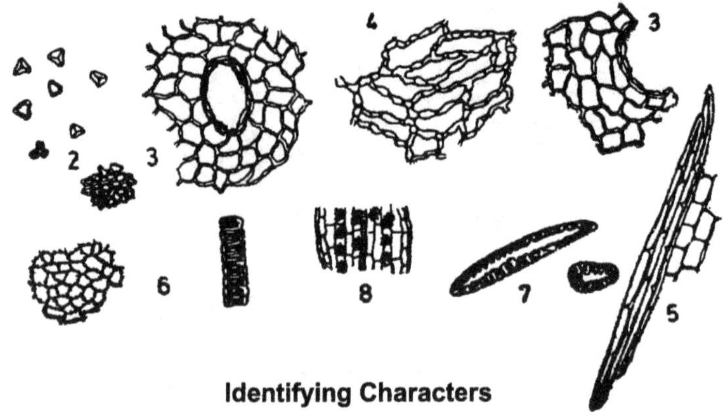

Identifying Characters

1. **Odour:** the typical aroma of the Eugenol.

2. **Pollen grains:** small, biconvex with rounded or triangular (angles not sharp) outline and a smooth exine. Masses of unripe pollen packets are also seen.

3. **Oil glands:** fragments of parenchyma containing entire or a portion of oil glands.

4. **Aerenchyma:** portion of loose parenchyma.

5. **Fibres:** sclerenchymatous fibres associated with parenchymatous cells.

6. **Anther:** fibrous layer of anther in surface view.

7. **Sclereids:** from the stalk, oval to subrectangular, thickened walls having numerous simple or branched pits.

8. **Calcium oxalate:** in the form of cluster crystals.

9. When starch is present then it is from Anthophylli (Mother Clove).

FLORES CHAMOMILE

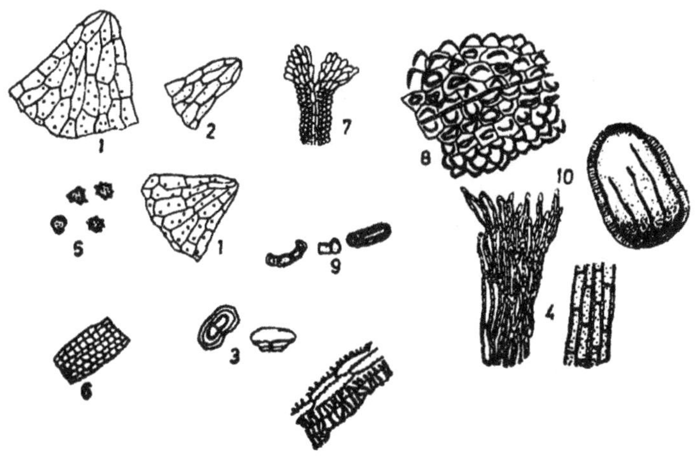

Identifying Characters

1. **Corolla:** numerous, fragments or entire apical pieces of corolla in surface view.

2. **Connective:** many apical pieces of connective of the filament.

3. **Trichomes:** many compositae type of glandular trichomes.

4. **Involucral bracts:** fragments showing sclerenchymatous cells with pitted thickenings.

5. **Pollen grains:** spiny with 3 ridges and furrows.

6. **Filament:** fragments of the epidermis of the filament in surface view.

7. **Stigma:** papillose and bifid.

8. **Ray florets:** papillose in nature.

9. **Stone cells:** from the basal region of the ovary.

10. **Ovary:** bulging like a balloon, transparent and on the walls of the concave-convex ovary are seen mucilaginous ribs or scales.

FLORES CINA (SANTONICA)

Artemisia cina (Berg) Willkomm.   Compositae

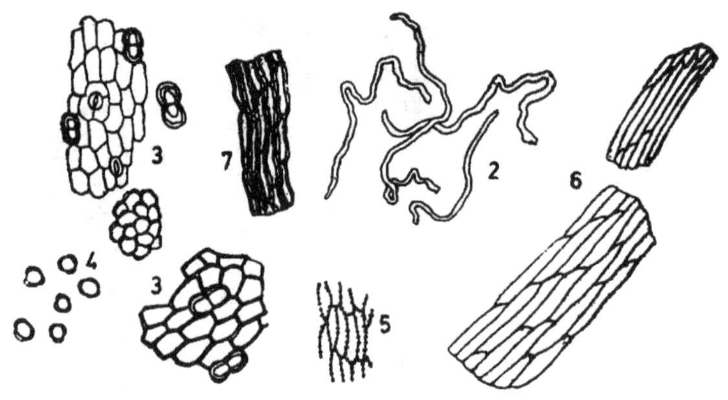

Identifying Characters

1. **Trichomes:** numerous, both covering and glandular.

2. **Covering trichomes:** worm shaped hairs or trichomes appear like that of cotton fibres seen through a microscope.

3. **Glandular trichomes:** compositae type, occur either single or in groups on the bracts and are particularly abundant on the outer epidermis of the central region.

4. **Pollen grains:** abundant, small sized, spherical with three ridges and three furrows. Groups of unripe pollen form pollen packets.

5. **Anther:** fibrous layer of the anther showing pits in surface view.

6. **Bract:** represented in fragments showing characteristic elongated cells.

7. **Sclereids:** from the central region of bracts.

FLORES PYRETHRI (PYRETHRUM)

Chrysanthemum cinerariifolium Vis.   Compositae

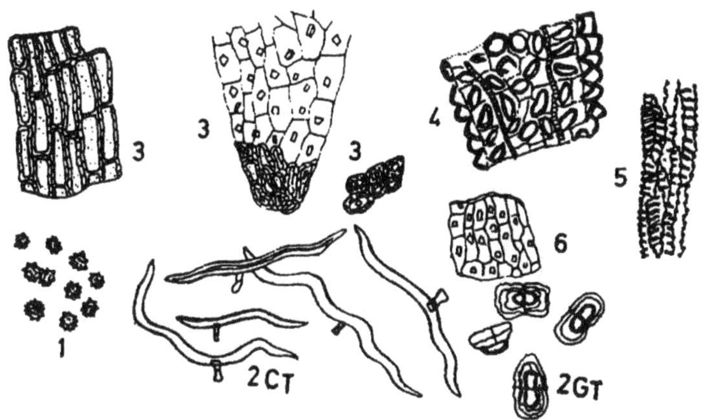

Identifying Characters

1. **Pollen grains:** globular with distinct furrows and ridges.

2. **Trichomes:** both covering and glandular type.

   Covering trichomes: entire or fragments of covering trichomes appearing in the form of the letter 'T'.

   Glandular trichomes: typical compositae type of glandular trichomes.

3. **Bracts:** groups of sclerenchymatous cells of the bract containing calcium oxalate prisms. The base of the bracts shows some typical sclereids.

4. **Corolla:** papillate in nature.

5. **Anther:** fibrous layer of anther.

6. **Calyx :** apical portion showing some isolated prisms.

FRUCTUS ANISI

Pimpinella anisum L.   Umbelliferae

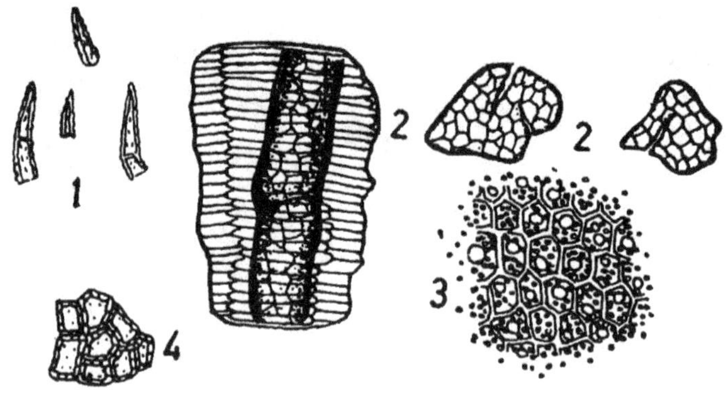

Identifying Characters

1. **Trichomes:** only covering trichomes – unicellular, short, blunt, conical and warty, emerging from the epidermis of the pericarp (epicarp).

2. **Endocarp:** fragments of endocarp on which yellow bands or zones of oil (vittae) are seen.

3. **Endosperm:** portions of endosperm containing oil globules and aleuroue grains which are small and most of them contain a rosette crystal of calcium oxalate.

4. **Stone cells:** not very common, occur in groups, pitted, rectangular with large lumen.

FRUCTUS CAPSICI (CAPSICUM)

Capsicum minimum Roxb   Solanaceae

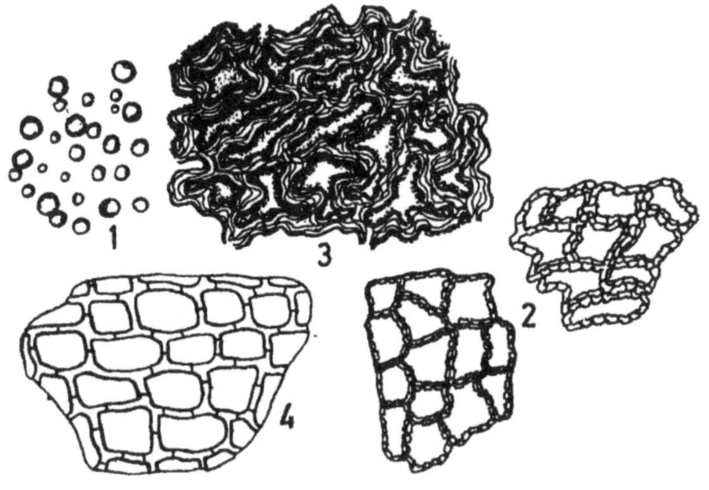

Identifying Characters

1. **Oil globules:** abundant and red coloured.

2. **Sclereids:** from the endocarp (in surface view), evenly thickened and pitted.

3. **Epidermis of the Testa:** (in surface view) highly convoluted, unevenly thickened and yellowish green in colour.

4. **Epicarp:** brown fragments of epicarp in surface view; cells are unevenly thickened and are polygonal to elongated.

FRUCTUS CARDAMOMI

Elettaria cardamomum White et Maton   Zingiberaceae

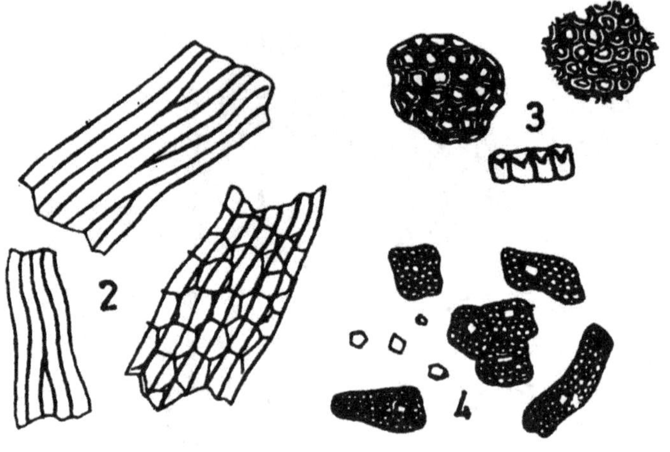

Identifying Characters

1. **Odour:** characteristic sweet aroma.

2. **Epidermal cells:** cells of the epidermis of testa are associated with a layer of oil cells. Epidermal cells are colourless to light yellow, straight walled and running almost parallel to each other.

3. **Sclerenchyma:** fragments of red to orange coloured sclerenchyma of the testa, individual cells of which are cylindrical and elongated in side view and polygonal in surface view, containing a nodule of silica.

4. **Perisperm:** of thin walled cells, colourless, granular and contains starch and also prisms of calcium oxalate.

Note: Cardamom though fruit, only seed characters are furnished here.

FRUCTUS CARVI (CARAWAY)

Carum carvi L.   Umbelliferae

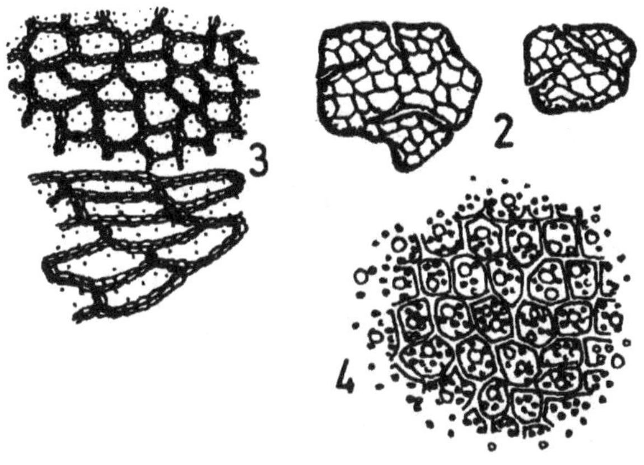

Identifying Characters

1. **Odour:** characteristic aroma.

2. **Vittae:** numerous yellow fragments composed of thin walled cells; because of the fine cracks, the fragments appear as broken glass pieces.

3. **Sclereids:** group of sclereids from the mesocarp.

4. **Endosperm:** large portions of endosperm with oil globules and aleurone grains with microsphenoidal crystals of calcium oxalate.

FRUCTUS CORIANDRI

Coriandrum sativum L.   Umbelliferae

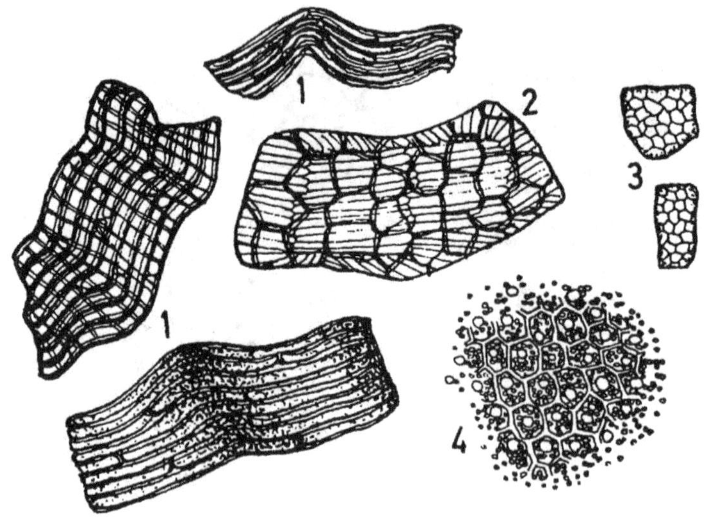

Identifying Characters

1. **Sclerenchymatous layer:** groups of   fusiform fibres of sclerenchyma running wavy and at times crossing with each other or with thin walled lignified cells of the mesocarp.

2. **Endocarp:** fragments of parquetry arrangement of thin walled lignified cells with the polygonal cells of mesocarp.

3. **Vittae:** few brown fragments of vittae.

4. **Endosperm:** fragments of endosperm with aleurone grains and oil globules.

FRUCTUS DILL (INDIAN DILL)

Anethum sowa Kurz.   Umbelliferae

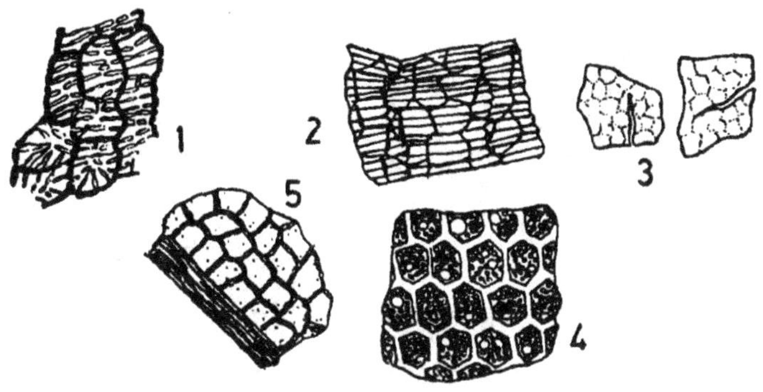

Identifying Characters

1. **Mesocarp:** parenchymatous cells of the mesocarp showing reticulate thickening.

2. **Endocarp:** parquetry arrangement is seen in surface view.

3. **Vittae:** with fine cracks like that on a broken glass.

4. **Endosperm:** presence of oil globules and aleurone grains.

5. **Sclereids:** many fragments of mesocarp each containing groups of stone cells. Each stone cell of a group is almost rectangular with pitted walls.

FRUCTUS FOENICULI (FENNEL)

Foeniculum vulgare Mill.   Umbelliferae

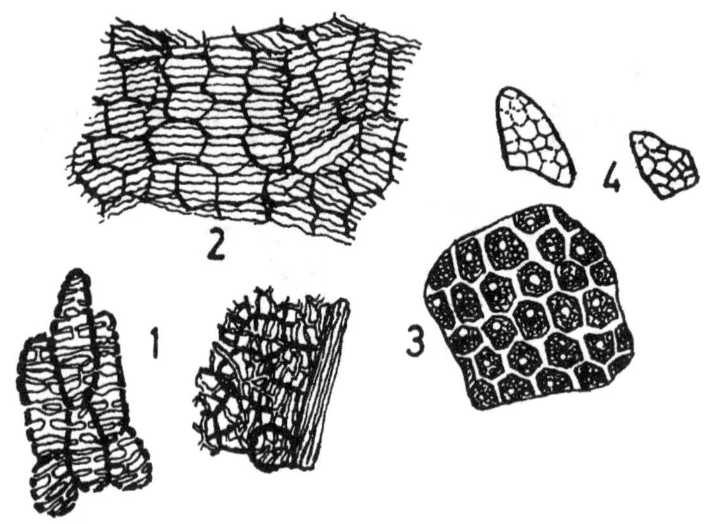

Identifying Characters

1. **Mesocarp:** lignified and reticulate nature of the parenchyma.
   Attention: Fructus Dill.

2. **Endocarp:** cells showing parquetry arrangement.

3. **Endosperm:** polyhedral, thick walled cells containing aleurone grains, minute calcium oxalate crystals and oil globules.

4. **Vittae:** many in the form of yellowish brown fragments.

5. **Odour:** characteristic sweet aroma.

FRUCTUS PIPERIS

Piper nigrum L.   Piperaceae

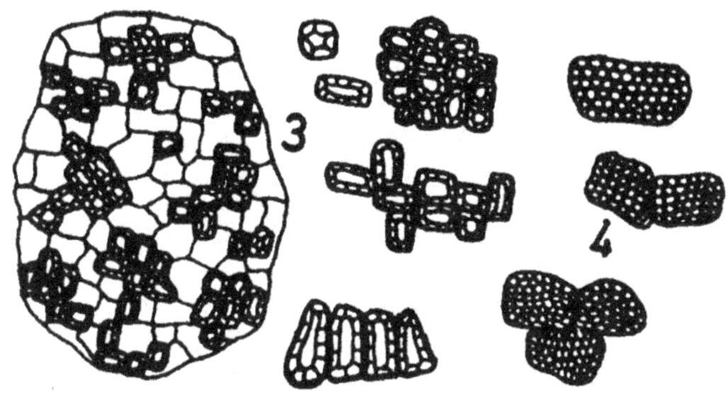

Identifying Characters

1. **Odour:** characteristic aroma; with pungent taste.

2. **Colour:** powder emits a yellow colouration on treating with Chloral hydrate.

3. **Stone cells:** groups of stone cells, nearly isodiametric with intercellular-space like – unthickened portions (simple pores?) in surface view. In sideview, some stone cells (from endocarp) appear as a row of 'beaker' shaped thick walled cells.

4. **Starch grains:** numerous, mostly in polyhedral masses. One should not confuse these polyhedral starchy masses to the perisperm fragments of Fructus **Cardamomi**.

SEMEN ARECA

Areca catechu L.   Palmae

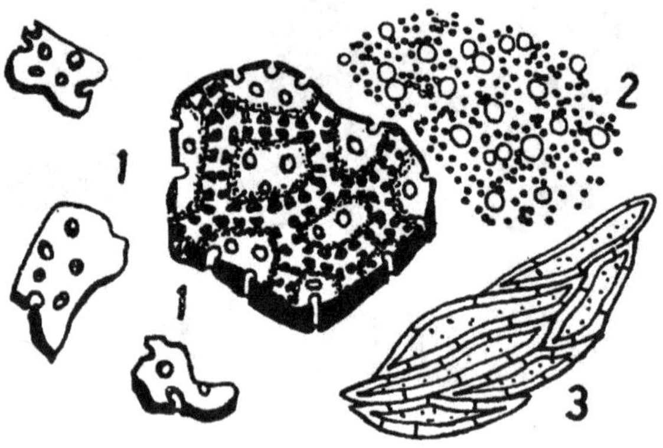

Identifying Characters

1. **Endosperm:** abundant fragments of characteristic endosperm cells. These cells are grey in colour, heavily thickened, porous and coarsely pitted.

2. **Oil globules:** large amount of oil globules and aleurone grains all over the slide, thus imparting a yellow colouration.

3. **Stone cells:** evenly thickened stone cells from the testa.

4. **Chemical test:** Ferric chloride solution on contact with the cell contents of the powder gives a greenish-black colouration (test for condensed tannins).

5. **Negative character:** absence of starch.

SEMEN COFFEAE (COFFEE)

Coffea arabica L.   Rubiaceae

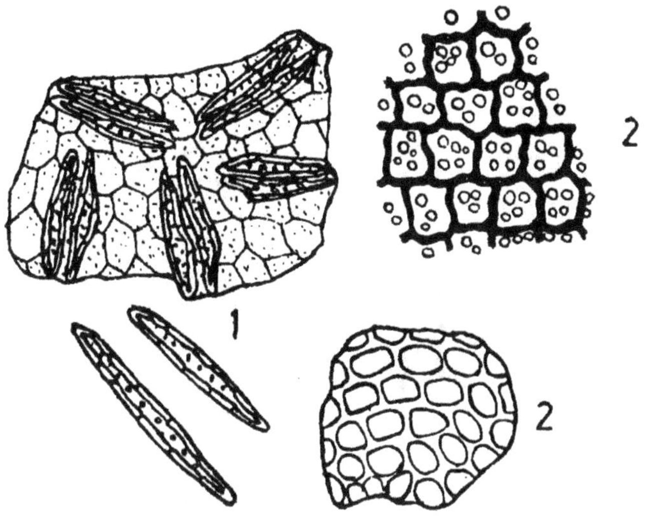

Identifying Characters

1. **Stone cells:** groups of yellow coloured stone cells are the characteristic feature of coffee powder. Each stone cell is linear, elongated with pits both on the wall and as well on the surface. These stone cells are found in the outer most skin of the coffee seed.

2. **Endosperm cells:** these are of two types; the ones near the margin are thick but smooth walled with no intercellular spaces. The others from the central part are numerous and show thick but convoluted walls, also without any intercellular spaces. Both show many oil globules.

Note: So as to get good clarity, it is better to boil the powder a couple of times in Chloral hydrate.

SEMEN COLCHICI

Colchicum autumnale L.

C. luteum Baker

Liliaceae

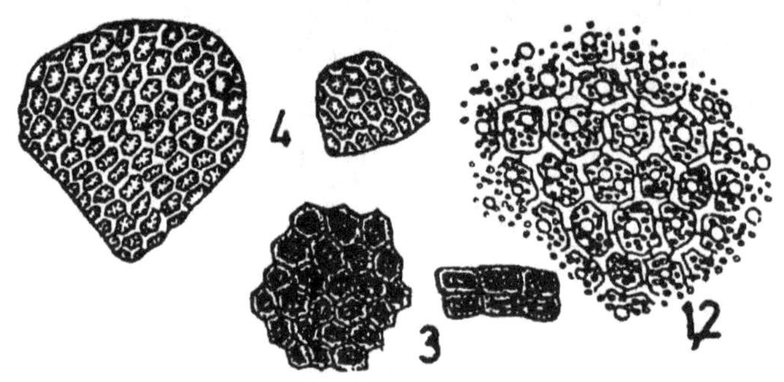

Identifying Characters

1. **Oil globules:** abundant and greyish in colour.

2. **Endosperm:** fragments of endosperm – parenchyma show characteristic pitted (porous) walled cells containing fixed oil and aleurone grains.

3. **Pigment layer:** brownish pigment layer in fragments.

4. **Testa:** characteristic fragments of brownish epidermis.

5. **Negative character:** absence of starch.

SEMEN ISPAGHULA

Plantago ovata Forsk   Plantaginaceae

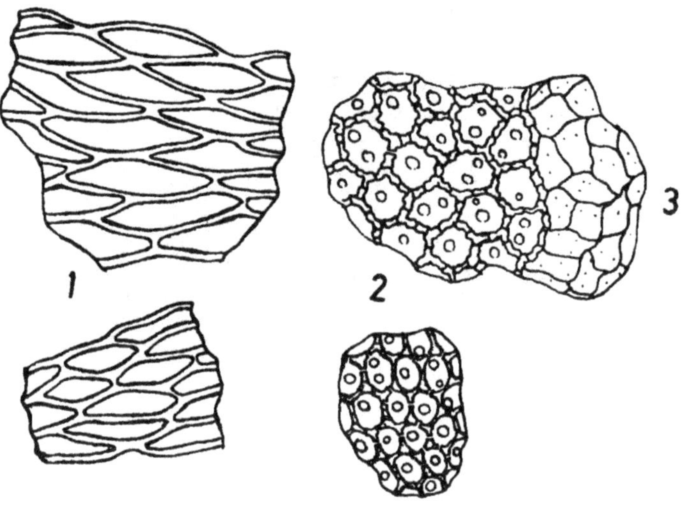

Identifying Characters

1. **Epidermis:** thick walled, transparent, polyhedral to tangentially elongated cells of the testa containing mucilage.

2. **Endosperm:** fragments of endosperm in surface view showing thickened cell walls with numerous pits.

3. **Testa:** a portion of testa containing yellow pigment layer associated with pitted cells of the endosperm.

4. **Chemical test:** solution of Ruthenium Red stains the mucilage pink.

SEMEN LINI (LINSEED)

Linum usitatissimum L.   Linaceae

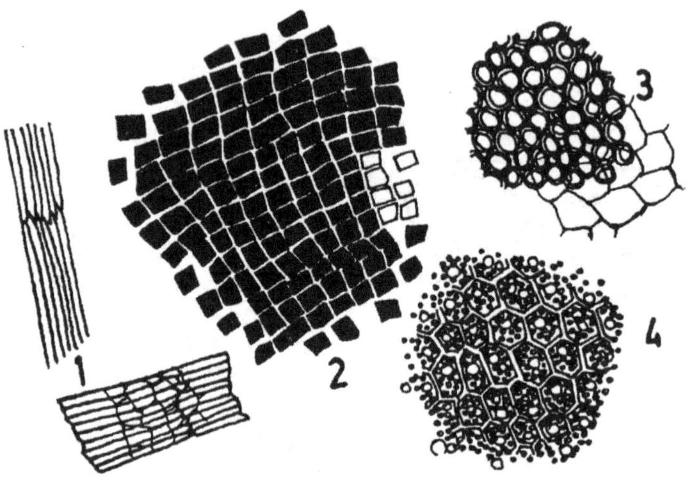

Identifying Characters

1. **Sclerenchymatous fibres of the testa:** these yellow coloured fibres consist of the slender, longitudinally stretched cells. Individual member of one group of fibres gets interwoven with a member from the successive group. At times these fibres cross the thin parenchymatous cells of the nutritive layer.

2. **Pigment layer:** fragments of the pigment layer of the testa consisting of square cells with orange brown mass, act as characteristic feature of linseed powder (blocks like that of Cadbury chocolate). The walls of these cells are pitted.

3. **Sub-epidermis:** fragments of rounded collenchymatous sub-epidermal cells in association with polygonal epidermal cells (surface view).

4. **Aleurone grains:** cells of the embryo and endosperm contain aleurone grains and fatty oil drops.

5. **Negative characters:** absence of starch and calcium oxalate crystals.

SEMEN MYRISTICAE (NUTMEG)

Myristica fragrans Houttuyn

Myristicaceae

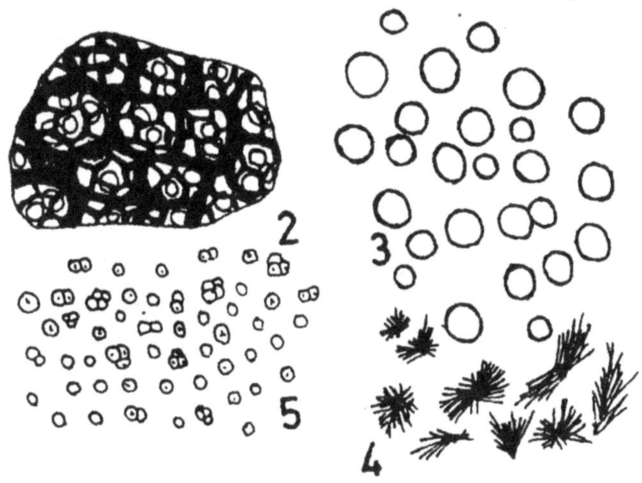

Identifying Characters

1. **Odour:** characteristic aroma.

2. **Oil cells:** big oil cells in brown perisperm fragments.

3. **Oil globules:** very big oil drops and numerous droplets.

4. **Fat-crystals:** crystalline groups of fat in the form of bunches of small needles (one can see these bushy needles only after sufficient cooling of the chloral hydrate preparation).

   Attention: Radix **Ipecac** and Bulbus **Scillae** (acicular raphides).

5. **Starch grains:** abundant, simple (spherical) and compound (2-8).

SEMEN STROPHANTHI

Strophanthus gratus Wall. et Hook   Apocynaceae

Strophanthus kombe Oliv.

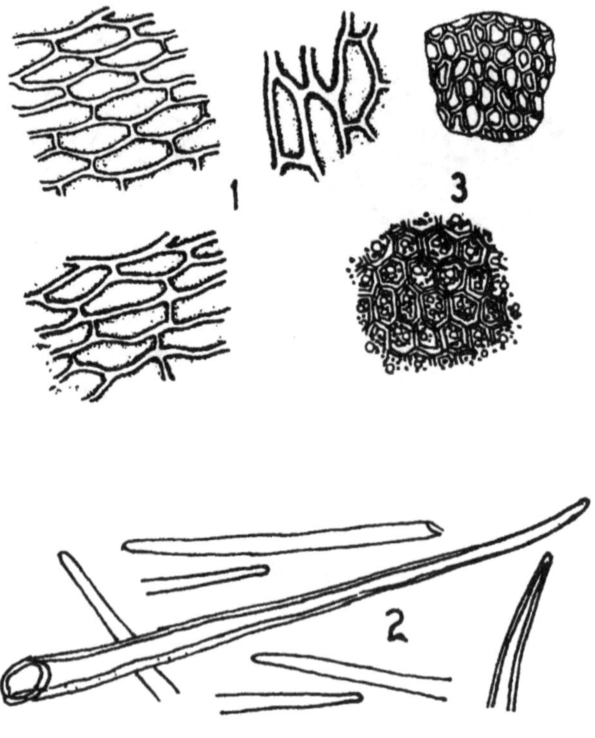

Identifying Characters

1. **Epidermis:** oval lignified thick walled characteristic epidermal cells either entire or in fragments but in groups.

2. **Trichomes:** lignified covering trichomes are present only in *S. kombe* and NOT in *S. gratus* (not shown in the diagram).

   Attention: Semen **Strychni.**

3. **Oil globules and Aleurone grains:** present in parenchyma of the cotyledons and endosperm.

SEMEN STRYCHNI (NUX VOMICA)

Strychnos nux-vomica L.   Loganiaceae

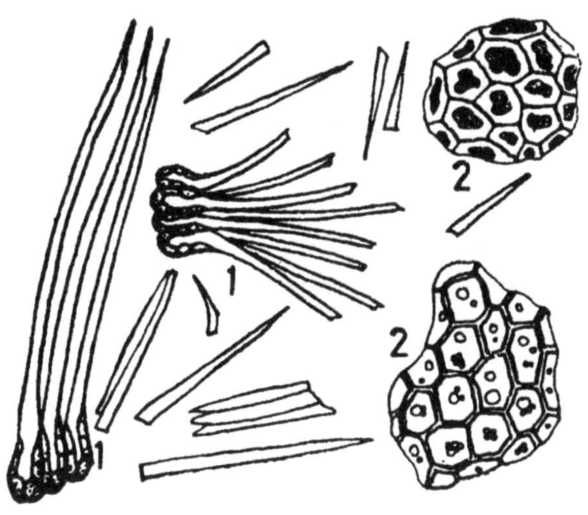

Identifying Characters

1. **Trichomes:** entire or fragments of lignified trichomes in abundance. At times the 'retort' shaped basal region of these trichomes can be seen in groups arising from common stock (the fragments of trichomes may appear as rod like crystals).

   Attention: Semen **Strophanthi**.

2. **Endosperm:** abundant fragments of endosperm cells whose walls are thickened.

3. **Negative character:** absence of starch.

HERBA CANNABIS (INDIAN HEMP)

Cannabis sativa L.   Cannabinaceae

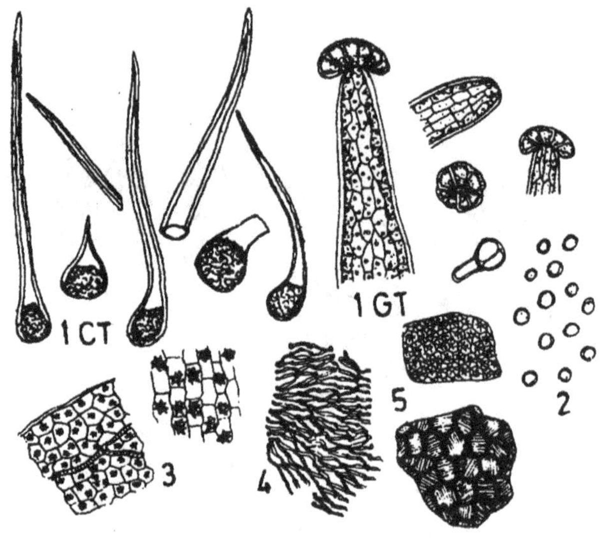

Identifying Characters

1. **Trichomes:** numerous, both covering and glandular.

   Covering trichomes: unicellular, rigid, slightly curved, pointed at one end and the other basal end is enlarged and contains cystolith (dagger shaped).

   Glandular trichomes: these are of two types – one with a multiseriate and multicellular tongue shaped stalk with a globular, multicellular head and the other with a short one-celled stalk and 8 celled head.

2. **Pollen grains:** simple, rounded and numerous.

3. **Calcium oxalate:** in the form of small cluster crystals, present in the bracteoles and stems as well (almost like that in Folia **Stramonii**).

4. **Parenchyma:** characteristic parenchymatous tissue of the wall of the ovary.

5. **Pericarp:** portion of brown sclerenchymatous layer of epicarp (in surface view).

HERBA EPHEDRA

Ephedra gerardiana (Wall.) Stapf.   Gnetaceae

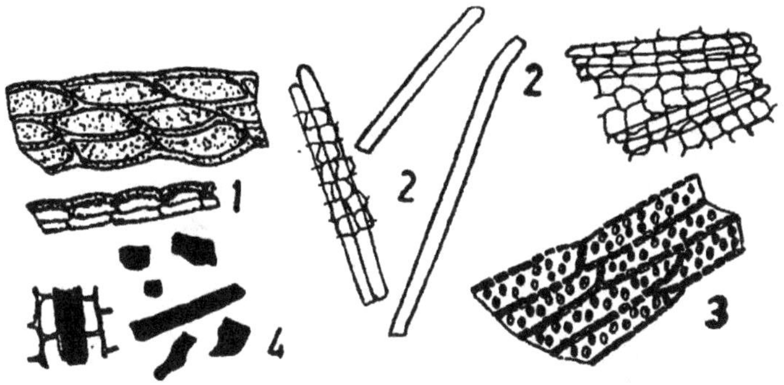

Identifying Characters

1. **Epidermis:** fragments of epidermal cells whose outer walls are ridged.

2. **Fibres:** both lignified and non-lignified fibres of uniform thickness, long, slender and cylindrical (like glass rods) appear either entire or in fragments.

3. **Wood elements:** consisting of only tracheids with bordered pits.

4. **Brownish matter:** abundant and possess regular shape and form. They originate from pith.

HERBA KALMEGH

Andrographis paniculata Nees.   Acanthaceae

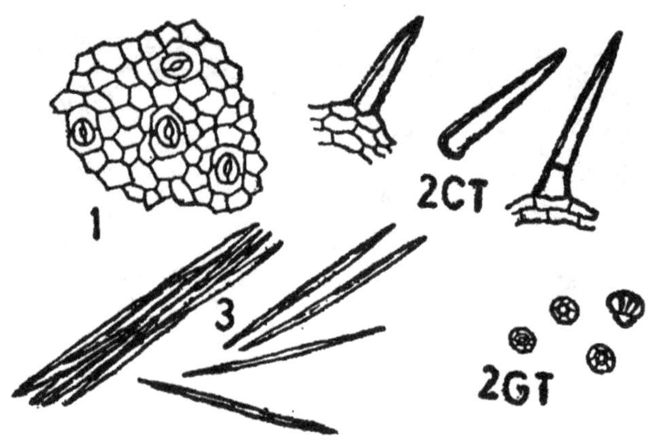

Identifying Characters

1. **Stomata:** Caryophyllaceous or diacytic type (the other examples are Folia **Mentha** and Folia **Vasaka**).

2. **Trichomes:** both glandular and covering trichomes are met with.

    Covering trichomes: one to three celled with a blunt apex, rough surface and with a slightly wavy margin.

    Glandular trichomes: with an unicellular stalk and a disc shaped head (seen both in side view as well in surface view).

3. **Fibres:** thin, long and slender fibres also called as acicular fibres.

ALOES

Aloe species   Liliaceae

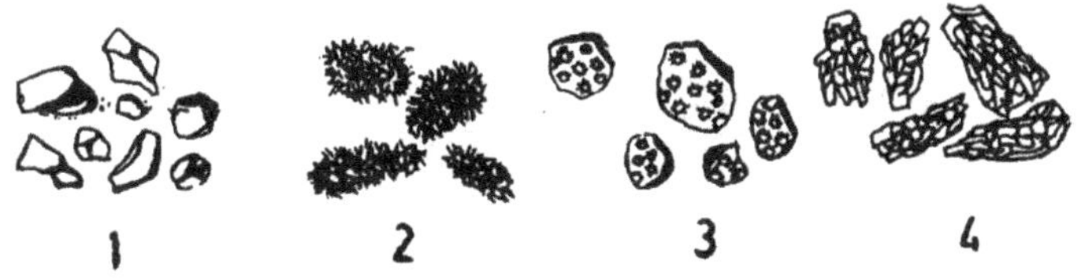

Identifying Characters

Note: preparations are to be made in Lactophenol mount.

1. **Cape Aloes:** fragments of transparent, shining, irregular crystalline bodies (resemble the finecracks of a broken glass).

2. **Curacao Aloes:** groups of prisms or fine needles.

3. **Zanzibar Aloes:** represented by irregularly embedded masses with sphaerite like appearances.

4. **Socotra Aloes:** groups of prisms aggregate to form irregular masses.

ERGOT OF RYE

Claviceps purpurea Tulasne.   *on Secale cereale* L.
(Hypocreaceae) Ascomycetes   Graminae

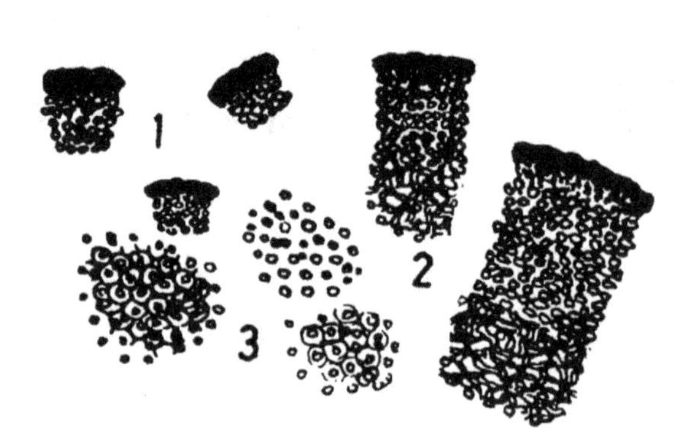

Identifying Characters

1. **Outer covering:** fragments of violet coloured cuticle (?).

2. **Hyphae:** thick walled hyphae (pseudoparenchyma) from the peripheral region of the sclerotium. The hyphae from the central region are losely interwoven and therefore difficult to see in the disintegrated tissue.

3. **Oil globules:** from the pseudoparenchyma.

AMYLUM MANIHOT
(TAPIOCA STARCH)

Source: *Manihot esculenta* Crantz.   Euphorbiaceae

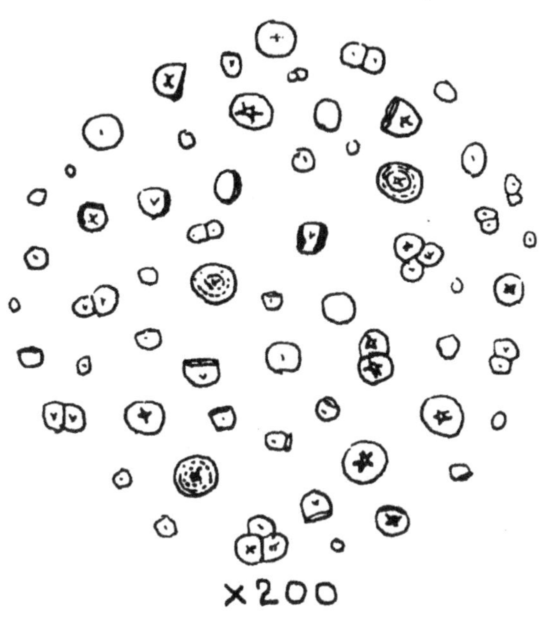

Identifying Characters

1. **Nature:** both simple and compound (2 – 3 components).

2. **Size:** 5 to 30 microns in diameter.

3. **Shape:** individual granules are rounded to spherical.

4. **Hilum:** central hilum is large and very often stellate.

5. **Striations:** some of the granules may show concentric striations.

57

AMYLUM MARANTAE
(ARROWROOT STARCH)

Source: *Maranta arundinacea* L.   Marantaceae

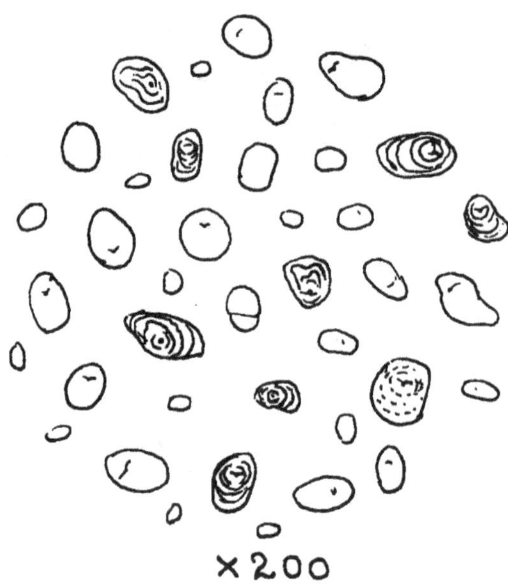

Identifying Characters

1. **Nature:** simple.

2. **Size:** vary in size from 7 – 75 microns.

3. **Shape:** vary in form from oval to ellipsoidal and some may even be pear shaped.

4. **Hilum:** the slightly eccentric hilum resembles the wings of a flying bird.

5. **Striations:** are often seen clearly.

AMYLUM MAYDIS
(MAIZE STARCH – CORN STARCH)

Source: *Zea mays* L.   Graminae

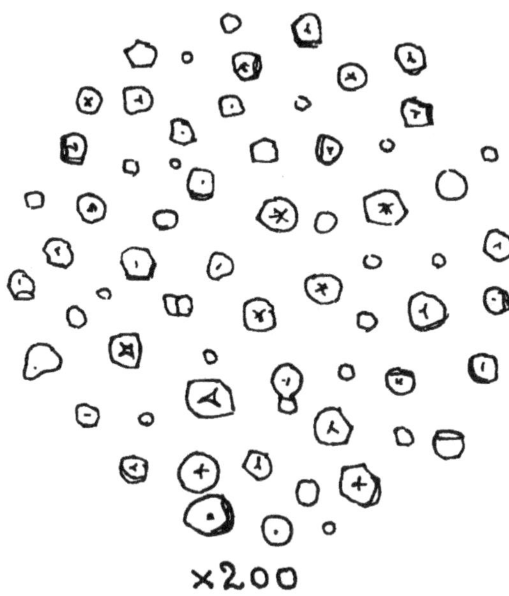

Identifying Characters

1. **Nature:** simple and compound.

2. **Size:** measure from 2 to 32 microns.

3. **Shape:** they are polyhedral to subspherical.

4. **Hilum:** distinct, stellate or star shaped.

5. **Striations:** not visible.

AMYLUM ORYZAE (RICE STARCH)

Source: *Oryza sativa* L.   Graminae

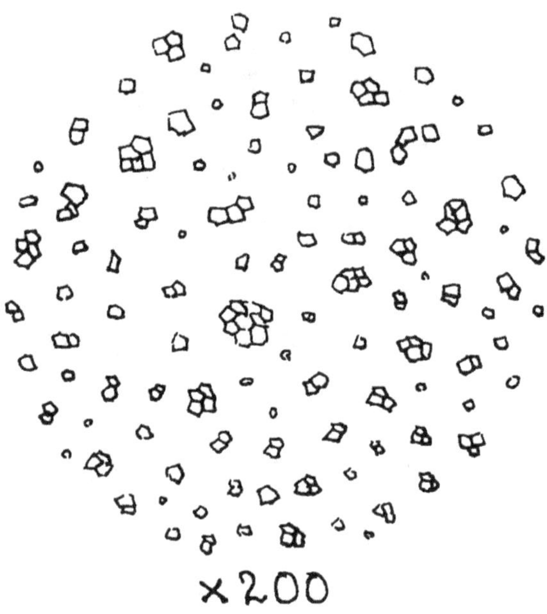

Identifying Characters

1. **Nature:** both simple and compound.

2. **Size:** very small and measure from 2 to 10 microns.

3. **Shape:** besides the polyhedral, angular, simple individual grains, there appear groups of such granules still within the outline of endosperm cells.

4. **Hilum:** not visible.

5. **Striations:** not visible.

AMYLUM SOLANI (POTATO STARCH)

Source: *Solanum tuberosum* L.   Solanaceae

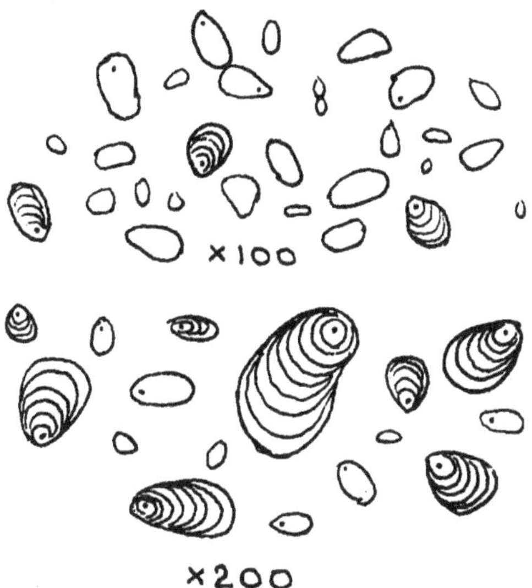

Identifying Characters

1. **Nature:** although most of the granules are simple, there are a few compound ones with 2 to 3 components.

2. **Size:** varies from 5 to 100 microns in length.

3. **Shape:** granules of the potato have a characteristic form which is oval to subspherical.

4. **Hilum:** not clearly seen but lies eccentric.

5. **Striations:** very clear.

AMYLUM TRITICI (WHEAT STARCH)

Source: *Triticum aestivum* L.   Graminae

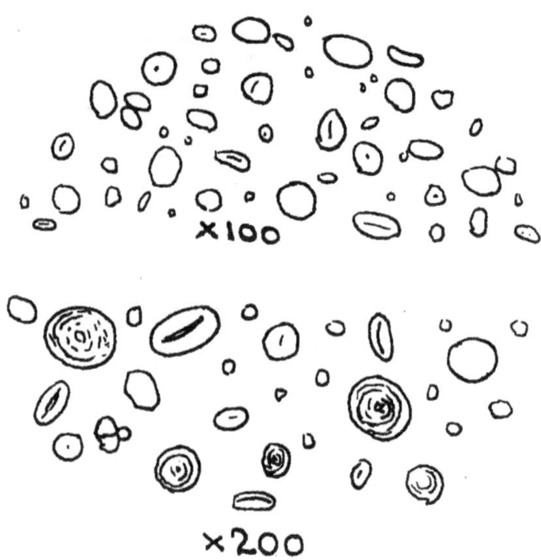

Identifying Characters

1. **Nature:** largely simple.

2. **Size:** two distinct size ranges are met with; the small ones measure from 2 to 9 microns and the bigger ones measure from 20 to 45 microns.

3. **Shape:** the bigger ones appear oval to spherical.

4. **Hilum:** seen as a shining line in side view.

5. **Striations:** they do show faint striations.

BIBLIOGRAPHY

Pharmacopoeia of India: Government of India Publication (1966).

British Pharmacopoeia: General Medical Council Publication, The Pharmaceutical Press, 17 Bloomsbury Square, London (1963).

Powdered Vegetable Drugs: B. P. Jackson and D. W. Snowdon; American Elsevier Publishing Company Inc. (1968).

Indian Pharmaceutical Codex: B. Mukerji, C. S. I. R. Publication, 1 (1953).

Lehrbuch der Pharmakognosie: E. Stahl, Gustav Fischer Verlag, Stuttgart (1962).

Chromatographische and Mikroskopische Analyse von Drogen: E. Stahl, Gustav Fischer Verlag, Stuttgart (1970).

Teenalyse: L. Horhammer, Springer Verlag, Berlin (1970).

Hagers Handbuch Der Pharmazeutischen Praxis: P. H. List and L. Horhammer, Springer Verlag, Berlin Heidelberg, 3 (1971).

Text Book of Pharmacognosy: T. E. Wallis, J & A Churchill Ltd., London 104 Gloucester Place, W. 1 (1955).

Text Book of Practical Pharmacognosy: B. E. Hebert and K. W. Ellery Bailliere, Tindall and Cox, London, 7 and 8 Henrietta Street (1948).